# FOOD CHOICES
## Eating for Health

**Mary Jo Tuckwell, R.D., MPH**

Family Health Center Nutritionist
St. Francis-Mayo Family Practice
Residency Program
LaCrosse, Wisconsin

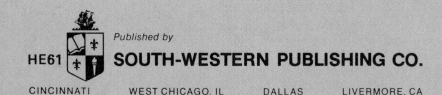

Published by

HE61 **SOUTH-WESTERN PUBLISHING CO.**

CINCINNATI WEST CHICAGO, IL DALLAS LIVERMORE, CA

**Consulting Editor:**

Theodora Faiola Priest, Ed. D.
Administrator, Marin County Office of Education,
    Vocational and Occupational Programs
San Rafael, California

Copyright © 1988
by South-Western Publishing Co.
Cincinnati, Ohio

ISBN: 0-538-32610-7

Library of Congress Catalog Number: 85-61352

1 2 3 4 5 6 7 8 Ki 3 2 1 0 9 8 7

*Printed in the United States of America*

# PREFACE

This is an invitation to explore a very personal subject—food choice and your health. Technological and social changes have created a marketplace of endless food choices. However, the foods available differ considerably in nutritional value, cost, and time and skill required for preparation. Selecting a healthful diet has become a challenge often requiring trade-offs between these factors. Food choice is a personal decision with individual as well as social consequences.

In a information-based society, the ability to collect, evaluate, and use information effectively is an essential consumer skill. Today both young men and women are frequently responsible for food purchasing and preparation. In a very practical sense, application of food and nutrition knowledge is a survival skill in our complex society. This text is designed to equip young adults with the food and nutrition knowledge needed to make informed decisions and recognize the consequences of those choices. The study of human nutrition relies on knowledge gained from biological, social, and economic sciences. Thus, this text is multidisciplinary in approach and may be a useful resource in more than one subject area.

To focus on the personal nature of food choice, readers are asked to identify how nutrition knowledge can benefit them. The text is divided into three skill-building sections. The first section, "Building Your Nutrition Knowledge," is intended to develop a basic understanding of nutrition as a science. Recognizing the scientific basis for the body's nutritional needs enables a consumer to appreciate the variety of foods needed for a healthful diet. The content of section one lends itself to studies in biological science, health, and home economics.

Interest in nutrition is captured by making the topic relevant to the reader. Themes that appeal to young adults are body image, health and fitness, and consumer issues of food cost and safety. The second section, "Making Informed Decisions," includes chapters on wellness, weight control, physical performance, identifying nutrition fallacies, and food production, food processing, and food safety. In this section readers apply nutrition knowledge to real-life issues. Chapters in this section may be suited to classes in health, physical education, home economics, agriculture, and consumer economics.

The last section of the text, "Healthy Eating Patterns," integrates scientific principles with the social science of eating behavior. Only by understanding the forces that influence food decisions can individuals make conscious choices to change behavior. In preparation for adult responsibilities, a separate chapter is devoted to meeting nutritional needs throughout the life-cycle. Readers are encouraged to identify changing nutrition needs with family members or friends of different ages. The closing chapter presents a current description of world hunger and efforts to meet food demands. The reader is challenged to use critical thinking skills in forming his or her own beliefs and actions on world food issues. The content lends itself to courses in home economics, values education, social studies, and consumer economics.

Each chapter opens with a nutrition scenario involving the reader in the application of the content to be presented. The beginning of each chapter features learner objectives that clearly highlight the points to be covered in the chapter. Key vocabulary words are italicized and defined. A glossary is also included. To reinforce concepts, the reader is asked to complete personal diet and lifestyle assessments. Numerous illustrations and tables are used to give emphasis or summarize major points. End-of-chapter questions are designed to assess recall and comprehension. A separate student activity guide features related application level learning experiences, including food preparation activities. The food composition table, Home and Garden Bulletin No. 72, is included in Appendix A as a reference for completing energy and nutrient analysis. Appendix C includes 90 recipes, selected to meet the U.S. Dietary Guidelines. These recipes may be used to demonstrate specific nutrition principles in a foods learning lab or serve as the reader's mini-cookbook for home use.

The accompanying instructor's manual serves as a curriculum and resource guide to supplement the text material. An objective content analysis is provided for use in matching the text material with individual course curriculum requirements. Teaching aids and current references are featured for each chapter. The manual includes answers to the end-of-chapter "Check Your Progress" section and student workbook activities. Sample chapter tests are provided as well.

To the readers of this text: A healthful diet can help you become all you desire to be. Choosing nutritious foods need not take the fun out of eating. As you read each chapter, be open to evaluating your diet and lifestyle. Studying nutrition will be easier and more meaningful if you relate chapter content to your own needs. Allow taste-testing of new foods to be an adventure. Keep track of the time and money saved as a food-smart consumer. Demonstrate your self-reliance by mastering basic food preparation skills. Discuss food and health issues with your family and friends. Remember, the more you know about food and nutrition the better prepared you will be to take care of yourself and others. Nutrition is a survival skill!

In conclusion, I would like to thank both Scherle Barth, M.S., R.D., and Pamela Van Zyl York, M.P.H., Ph.D., R.D., for their contributions to the manuscript of this text. I would also like to acknowledge the assistance of Susan Johnson-Leifer, R.D.

*Mary Jo Tuckwell*

# MEET THE AUTHOR

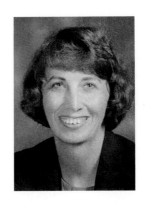

*Mary Jo Tuckwell*

Ms. Tuckwell is a registered dietitian and a nationally recognized nutrition educator. She obtained a Bachelor of Science degree in Dietetics from the University of Wisconsin–Stout and completed a dietetic internship and Master's degree in Public Health Nutrition at the University of California–Berkeley. Her skills as an educator have been developed through academic training in methods of teaching and curriculum development as well as through practical experience in a variety of formal and informal instructional settings.

Ms. Tuckwell has held positions as a public health nutritionist, college/university instructor, clinical dietitian, Extension nutrition specialist, and vocational project coordinator. Most notably she designed and implemented the Nutrition Education and Training Program for the Wisconsin Department of Public Instruction. Currently, Ms. Tuckwell is a nutritionist with the St. Francis–Mayo Family Practice Residency Program and Family Health Center in LaCrosse, Wisconsin.

Professional affiliations include the Society for Nutrition Education, American Dietetic Association, Wisconsin Dietetic Association, American Home Economics Association, Wisconsin Home Economics Association, American Public Health Association, Wisconsin Public Health Association, and Wisconsin Nutrition Council.

# CONTENTS

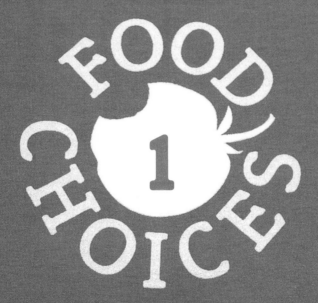

**FOOD CHOICES**

**1**

**BUILDING YOUR NUTRITION KNOWLEDGE**

1. Food: The Choices You Make
2. Your Need for Energy
3. Energy Plus
4. The Regulators
5. Nutritious Foods From Soup to Nuts

# FOOD: THE CHOICES YOU MAKE

Susan dreams of being a dancer. Feeling fit and looking great may help her dreams come true. Charlie is a member of the wrestling team. He needs to maintain his wrestling weight. Jennifer lives in an apartment and is trying to save money to attend college. How might these different goals influence their food choices?

In a marketplace filled with endless food choices, your knowledge and attitudes will be your guide. Food and nutrition awareness can help you reach your goals, too.

People have many reasons for learning more about nutrition. A mother-to-be wants to have the healthiest baby possible. A teenager diagnosed as diabetic struggles to understand and manage the disease. Parents, juggling careers and a family, need strength and stamina. Nutrition is a survival skill for today and tomorrow.

*Your objectives in this chapter will be to:*

- *Relate how nutrition knowledge may be of value to you*
- *Define nutrition as a science*
- *Identify the major classes of nutrients*
- *Explain the use of the Recommended Dietary Allowances*

## EATING . . . IT'S MORE THAN A PASTIME

Although eating is usually an enjoyable experience, it is much more than merely a pastime. A person's food choice today affects his or her health both now and in the future. However, many factors shape our food choices. Personal goals and values influence our attitudes and behavior about health and nutrition. How can developing your nutrition knowledge be of value to you?

**3**

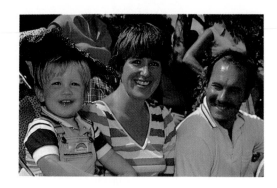

*Figure 1.1.* Today's food choices affect a person's health now and in the future.

## Building a Healthful Image

Being overweight is a physical and emotional health hazard, but compulsive dieting and being underweight are just as dangerous. Dull, dry hair and a poor complexion detract from physical appearance. A tired and irritable person sends negative messages about himself or herself to others. Your nutrition can make a difference in how you feel and look. A nutritious diet contributes to a radiant smile, smooth skin, muscular development, and desirable body weight. Whether your goal is to be a model or simply feel good about yourself, applying a few nutrition tips may work wonders.

## The Wellness Movement

Health is a vague term to most of us. As long as we feel good, we assume we are healthy. In fact, many people do not appreciate health until they become ill. But health means more than just the absence of illness. Many Americans are striving to achieve *wellness*. Wellness, both physical and emotional, depends on the prevention of disease. Prevention may include changes in life-style, since some personal decisions may increase your chance of illness or injury. For example, drinking alcohol and driving increase the chances of being involved in a car accident. Any injury sustained in this instance would be a visible and immediate result of personal behavior. However, not all life-style decisions have immediate consequences. Habits such as smoking or alcohol abuse place people at greater risk for long-term (chronic) diseases. Dietary factors have also been linked to the

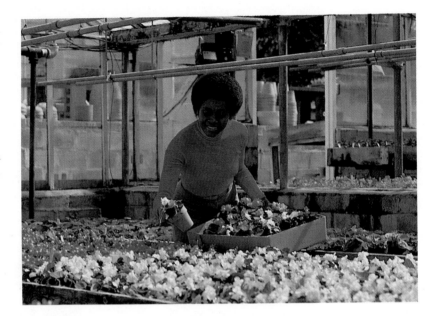

*Figure 1.2.*   A healthy body makes a person look good and feel good.

development of some chronic diseases including heart disease and certain forms of cancer. If you are interested in wellness, nutrition knowledge is a must.

## Achieving Physical Fitness

An athlete knows training is important to develop skill and physical fitness, but even with many hours of practice he or she may fall short of doing his or her best. A diet inadequate in energy or specific nutrients may hinder performance. Regardless of whether your physical exercise is for fun or competition good nutrition is essential, but beware of sports and fitness nutrition myths. Nutrition knowledge can help you judge the merits of special diet plans and products.

## Living on a Budget

Knowing nutrition facts is also a wise financial investment.

Managing to live on a budget is always a challenge. Did you know that food purchases may total as much as 16% to 30% of your income? Meat is often the most expensive item on the grocery list. Did you know protein can also be obtained from less expensive items

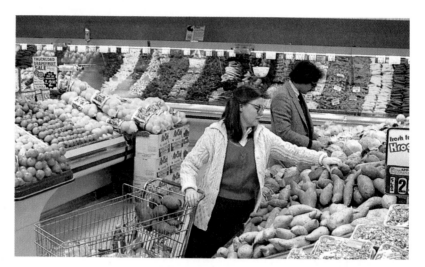

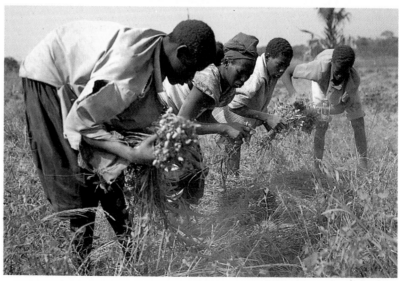

***Figure 1.3.*** All the many different foods a person eats make up his or her *diet*.

such as grains, dried peas and beans, seeds and nuts, and milk products? Convenience foods and ready-to-eat snacks are also very expensive per portion served. Planning to eat well on a budget means being a knowledgeable consumer.

### Nutrition Begins with Food Choice

Frequently people say, "I'm going on a diet." In popular conversation the word "diet" means avoiding or substituting certain foods, usually to achieve weight loss. Nutritionists refer to someone's *diet* as the collection of foods regularly consumed by an individual. Information on what is needed in a good diet is available from many sources. However, sometimes this information is conflicting, and deciding what nutrition advice to follow may be a confusing experience.

A nutritionally adequate diet may be built around a variety of foods. Can you plan a diet that is personally satisfying, nutritionally adequate, and economically feasible? These skills can be developed through practice and through an understanding of nutriton as a science.

## THE SCIENCE OF NUTRITION

*Nutrition* is the science of food and its use in the body. The study of nutrition is closely related to the fields of biology, biochemistry, physiology, agriculture, and food technology. As an applied science nutrition relies heavily on principles of sociology, psychology, and economics.

As with any science, the collection of nutrition facts evolves as theories are tested by scientists and researchers. To become a fact, the evidence gathered must be reproduced time after time with the same results. Because nutrition research is ongoing, not every question will have a right answer and wrong answer.

Throughout history people have held various ideas about the magical and medicinal powers of food. However, as a field of study, nutrition is comparatively young. During the 1800s and 1900s, chemists identified basic relationships among food, energy, and growth. In 1838 a substance containing nitrogen was identified in food. This substance was called protein. Through the years more of these components of foods were identified. Eventually in the early 1900s nutrition scientists were able to identify diseases caused by the lack of specific dietary components.

These essential dietary components became known as nutrients. *Nutrients* are chemical substances required for the proper functioning of the body. These nutrients as present in food must be separated and reduced to their most basic form to be of use in the body. Thus the study of nutrition also includes the processes by which the body obtains nutrients from food.

## Research: Discovering Relationships

Earlier nutrition research concentrated on identification of the essential components of food, the nutrients. Scientists have demonstrated that we need about 44 different nutrients for a healthy diet. Recent study has focused on the relationship between nutrients and exact human requirements for each nutrient. Today scientific concern for adequate nutrient intake has expanded to examining the relationship between diet and chronic disease; this relationship will be discussed in Chapter 6.

Use caution in applying what you read and hear about nutrition in the popular press. In an effort to bring nutrition information to

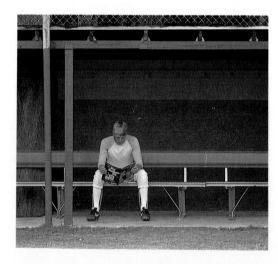

*Figure 1.4.* Nutrition information comes from many different—and sometimes contradictory—sources.

public attention, journalists may overstate research results. Increasing your nutrition knowledge will help you be more critical of the information that bombards you daily. Let's take a closer look at the body's need for nutrients.

# NUTRIENTS: AN OVERVIEW

Each nutrient plays a role in the body. Nutrients are responsible for supplying energy, providing materials for body growth and maintenance, and regulating body functions. Nutrients with similar functions are grouped together. The six major classes of nutrients are *water, carbohydrates, fats, proteins, vitamins,* and *minerals.* See Table 1.1.

## Water, Water Everywhere

The most abundant nutrient in food is water. Water is also the most critical nutrient for sustaining life. In fact, about two thirds of

### Table 1.1    Six Major Classes of Nutrients

| Nutrient Class | Functions |
| --- | --- |
| Water | Component of body fluids<br>Regulates body temperature<br>Transports nutrients and waste |
| Carbohydrates | Primary energy source |
| Fats | Concentrated energy source<br>Carry fat-soluble vitamins and essential fatty acids |
| Proteins | Provide building blocks for body tissue and compounds<br>Secondary energy source |
| Vitamins | Regulate body processes |
| Minerals | Regulate body processes |

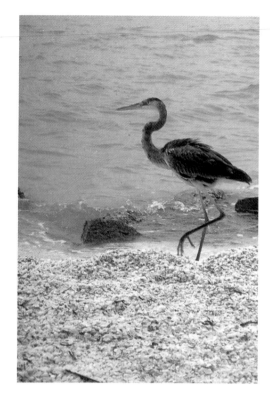

*Figure 1.5.* Water is absolutely essential to life.

the human body is water. Water is required for diluting and transporting other nutrients and waste products. It is also necessary for maintaining body temperature and for creating the coating for body joints. See Illustration 1.1.

## Energy: Power to Go and Grow

After the need for water has been satisfied, energy is of primary importance for the body's operation. Energy is needed to keep blood circulating, maintain body temperature, promote tissue growth and repair, and power body movements. The three nutrients capable of providing the body with energy are carbohydrates, fats, and proteins.

Most foods contain a mixture of each of these energy-providing nutrients. Some foods may be substantially higher in one nutrient than another. Therefore, foods are often classified by the

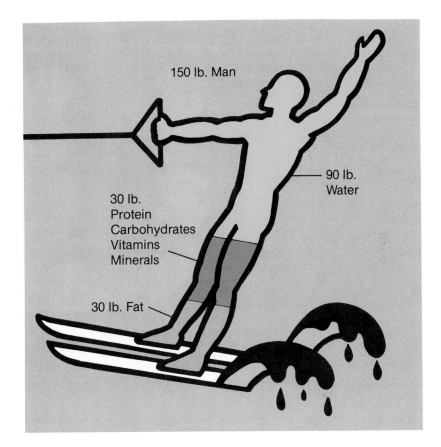

*Illustration 1.1.*
A person weighing
150 pounds has 90
pounds of water.

major nutrient(s) present. For example, bread is considered a carbohydrate food, yet it is also a source of fat and protein. A few foods, such as sugar and oil, contain only one energy nutrient. Sugar is a simple form of carbohydrate, while salad oil is a source of fat. Since foods differ in their nutrient content, they also provide varying amounts of energy. How to determine the energy value of food is explained in Chapter 3.

**The Preferred Fuel: Carbohydrates.** A *carbohydrate* is a substance composed of carbon, hydrogen, and oxygen atoms. In its simplest form its atoms are linked together to form a unit of *sugar.* Sugars are naturally present in such foods as milk, honey, fruit, and sugar cane. *Starch* is a more complex form of carbohydrate. Cereal

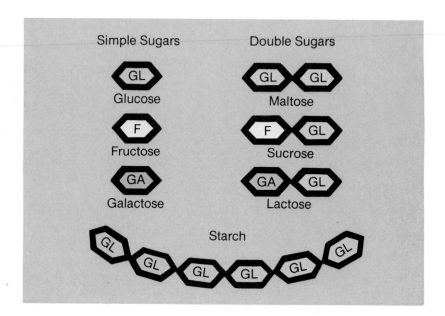

***Illustration 1.2.***
Forms of Carbohydrate.

grains such as wheat, rice, and corn are excellent sources of starch. *Glucose* is the end product of the body's digestive breakdown of starch and sugar. See Illustration 1.2. The brain and nervous system function most effectively when powered by glucose. How your body uses carbohydrates for energy is described in Chapter 3.

   Several other carbohydrates provide only dietary fiber. Humans cannot digest these carbohydrates; thus they cannot be used for energy. Nevertheless, they are recognized as valuable in keeping food and digestive waste products moving normally through the intestinal tract. Fiber is found in the outer covering of cereal grains, in stems and leaves of plants, and in skins of fruits and vegetables. See Illustration 1.3.

   ***A Pinch of Fat.*** *Fats* are carbon-containing substances that cannot be dissolved in water. A fat that is liquid at room temperature is called an *oil*. Most fat in our diet is composed of *triglycerides,*

***Illustration 1.3.***
Fiber: An Indigestible Carbohydrate.

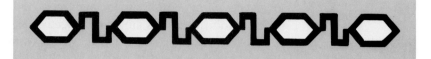

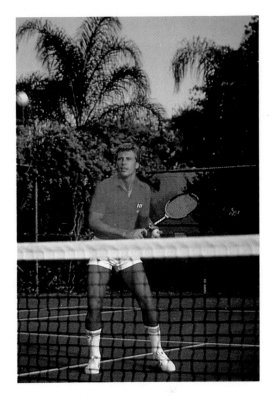

**Figure 1.6.** Carbohydrates are the favorite fuel of the brain and the body.

which consist of three fatty acids and glycerol. See Illustration 1.4. Because fats are carriers of certain vitamins, it is important to consume some fat in the diet. Determining how much fat consumption is healthy will be examined more closely in Chapter 6.

Fats are readily visible in such foods as butter, margarine, and vegetable oil. However, hidden sources of fat in whole milk, cheese, meat, and nuts also add to total fat intake.

**Illustration 1.4.** Triglycerides: Fatty Acid and Glycerol.

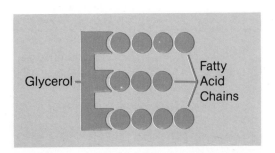

*Illustration 1.5.*
Proteins: Amino Acids
Linked Together.

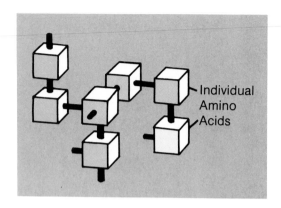

Individual
Amino
Acids

***Proteins: The Building Blocks.*** Although it may be used for energy, *protein* has a more important task: to build body tissue. Protein is composed of nitrogen-containing substances called *amino acids.* Your body can make some of the amino acids, whereas others must be obtained from food. In addition to building body cells, protein is necessary to make enzymes, maintain fluid levels, regulate acid/base balance, and produce hormones and antibodies. See Illustration 1.5.

Plant and animal foods vary greatly in amino acid composition. Different numbers of amino acids can be chemically arranged in endless combinations. For example, protein in beef muscle is entirely different from protein in corn. As you will see in Chapter 13, this fact is particularly important in the choice of foods to meet protein needs.

## Nutrients for Internal Control

***Vitamins.*** *Vitamins* are *organic,* or carbon-containing, compounds required in very small amounts to keep the body healthy. Vitamins regulate specific chemical reactions in the body. Vitamins cannot be broken down to provide energy. The diet must supply the needed vitamins as the body is unable to produce them in adequate quantities. To date, 13 vitamins have been identified as necessary to our health.

No one food contains all the vitamins a person needs. Some vitamins dissolve in water, while others will only mix with fat. Thus vitamins are generally classified as either *fat soluble* or *water soluble.*

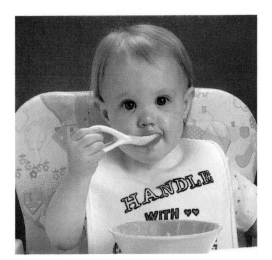

***Figure 1.7.*** Protein is needed to build body tissue.

Fat-soluble vitamins are stored by the body, whereas excess water-soluble vitamins are excreted. Because the body cannot store these water-soluble vitamins, it is important to consume water-soluble vitamins each day. See Illustration 1.6.

***Minerals.*** The term *minerals* refers to elements in their simple inorganic, or non-carbon-containing form. Currently 21 minerals are known to be needed by the body. Like vitamins, minerals do not provide energy. Minerals likewise regulate body reactions and are required in relatively small amounts.

***Illustration 1.6.*** Classification of Vitamins by Carrier in Which They Dissolve.

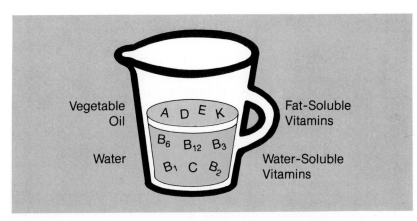

Minerals are widely distributed in the body. Minerals such as calcium and phosphorus function as structural materials in bones and teeth. Sodium and potassium control the flow of substances in and out of cells. Iron is needed to form *hemoglobin,* a substance that carries oxygen in the bloodstream. Other minerals form acids and bases, conduct nerve impulses, and link together to form organic molecules. The foods we eat vary greatly in mineral content.

# LIFELONG NEED FOR NUTRIENTS

Everyone, from a baby to a senior citizen, needs the same nutrients, but in different amounts. Factors that affect individual nutrient needs are *age, sex, body size,* and *activity level.* For example, teenagers are undergoing a rapid growth spurt. At the same time, they may be involved in high-energy activities such as sports, strenuous work, or dancing. It stands to reason that their need for certain nutrients and energy may be greater than that of an elderly person. Not only are older people often less physically active, but as we age the body's internal operations slow down. Thus the energy requirement for body maintenance decreases with age. However, conditions such as illness, fever, and burns can increase nutrient and energy needs. Other conditions such as pregnancy, breast-feeding, and stress also alter nutrient needs.

How much of each nutrient is needed to promote growth and maintain health? The United States government was particularly concerned about this question during the shortage of food in World War II. In 1943 a group of nutrition scientists met to develop nutrient intake recommendations. The recommendations were designed to ensure nutritional adequacy of meals for the military and the general public during the war.

Out of this initial need for guidelines, the *Recommended Dietary Allowances* (RDAs) were developed. National nutrition surveys conducted in the past 15 years have provided data on common nutritional problems in the United States. Particular concerns for the teenager are summarized in Table 1.2. Information gathered from all these sources helps scientists reevaluate human needs for nutrients on an ongoing basis. The process of conducting nutrition research will be discussed in detail in Chapter 9.

The RDAs represent levels of nutrient and energy intake

| **Table 1.2   Problem Nutrients in Teenage Diets** |
| --- |
| Iron |
| Calcium |
| Magnesium |
| Vitamin $B_6$ |

Source: United States Department of Agriculture, National Food Consumption Preliminary Report No. 2 (Washington, D.C.: United States Government Printing Office).

believed to be adequate for the nutritional needs of practically all healthy Americans. See Table 1.2. Note these recommendations are allowances, with a margin of safety built in above the minimum needs. The RDAs are updated as nutrition researchers discover new information. Nutrient allowances are specified in units of measure ranging from micrograms and milligrams to grams. Some vitamin levels are expressed in terms of their chemically active portion, such as retinol equivalents which are a measure of vitamin A activity.

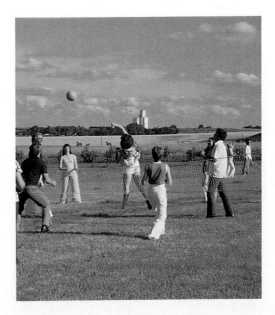

*Figure 1.8.*   Age, sex, body size, and activity level affect the amount of nutrients each individual needs.

## Table 1.3   Recommended Daily Dietary Allowances[a]

| | | Weight | | Height | | | Fat-Soluble Vitamins | | | Water-Soluble Vitamins | |
| --- | --- | --- | --- | --- | --- | --- | --- | --- | --- | --- | --- |
| | Age (years) | (kg) | (lb) | (cm) | (in) | Protein (g) | Vita-min A (μg RE)[b] | Vita-min D (μg)[c] | Vita-min E (mg α-TE)[d] | Vita-min C (mg) | Thia-min (mg) |
| Infants...... | 0.0-0.5 | 6 | 13 | 60 | 24 | kg×2.2 | 420 | 10 | 3 | 35 | 0.3 |
| | 0.5-1.0 | 9 | 20 | 71 | 28 | kg×2.0 | 400 | 10 | 4 | 35 | 0.5 |
| Children.... | 1-3 | 13 | 29 | 90 | 35 | 23 | 400 | 10 | 5 | 45 | 0.7 |
| | 4-6 | 20 | 44 | 112 | 44 | 30 | 500 | 10 | 6 | 45 | 0.9 |
| | 7-10 | 28 | 62 | 132 | 52 | 34 | 700 | 10 | 7 | 45 | 1.2 |
| Males....... | 11-14 | 45 | 99 | 157 | 62 | 45 | 1000 | 10 | 8 | 50 | 1.4 |
| | 15-18 | 66 | 145 | 176 | 69 | 56 | 1000 | 10 | 10 | 60 | 1.4 |
| | 19-22 | 70 | 154 | 177 | 70 | 56 | 1000 | 7.5 | 10 | 60 | 1.5 |
| | 23-50 | 70 | 154 | 178 | 70 | 56 | 1000 | 5 | 10 | 60 | 1.4 |
| | 51+ | 70 | 154 | 178 | 70 | 56 | 1000 | 5 | 10 | 60 | 1.2 |
| Females .... | 11-14 | 46 | 101 | 157 | 62 | 46 | 800 | 10 | 8 | 50 | 1.1 |
| | 15-18 | 55 | 120 | 163 | 64 | 46 | 800 | 10 | 8 | 60 | 1.1 |
| | 19-22 | 55 | 120 | 163 | 64 | 44 | 800 | 7.5 | 8 | 60 | 1.1 |
| | 23-50 | 55 | 120 | 163 | 64 | 44 | 800 | 5 | 8 | 60 | 1.0 |
| | 51+ | 55 | 120 | 163 | 64 | 44 | 800 | 5 | 8 | 60 | 1.0 |
| Pregnant........ | | | | | | +30 | +200 | +5 | +2 | +20 | +0.4 |
| Lactating........ | | | | | | +20 | +400 | +5 | +3 | +40 | +0.5 |

Source: Food and Nutrition Board, National Academy of Sciences, National Research Council, *Recommended Dietary Allowances,* ed. 9 (Washington, D.C.: National Academy Press, 1980).
[a]The allowances are intended to provide for individual variations among most normal persons as they live in the United States under usual environmental stresses. Diets should be based on a variety of common foods in order to provide other nutrients for which human requirements have been less well defined.
[b]Retinol equivalents. 1 retinol equivalent = 1 μg retinol or 6 μg β carotene.
[c]As cholecalciferol. 10 μg cholecalciferol = 400 IU of vitamin D.
[d]α-tocopherol equivalents. 1 mg d-α tocopherol = 1 α-TE.
[e]1 NE (niacin equivalent) is equal to 1 mg of niacin or 60 mg of dietary tryptophan.

RDAs are not requirements for individuals, but guidelines used by professionals for meal planning. Consuming less than two thirds of the RDA over a long period of time may increase the likelihood of nutrient *deficiency.* Similarly, consuming more than needed may produce a *toxic,* or harmful, effect. Examples of nutrient deficiency and toxicity are described in Chapter 4. For a consumer, determining the daily intake of nutrients is unrealistic and unnecessary. Under-

| Water-Soluble Vitamins | | | | | Minerals | | | | | |
|---|---|---|---|---|---|---|---|---|---|---|
| Ribo-flavin (mg) | Niacin (mg NE)[e] | Vita-min B$_6$ (mg) | Fola-cin[f] (µg) | Vitamin B$_{12}$ (µg) | Cal-cium (mg) | Phos-phorus (mg) | Mag-nesium (mg) | Iron (mg) | Zinc (mg) | Iodine (µg) |
| 0.4 | 6 | 0.3 | 30 | 0.5[g] | 360 | 240 | 50 | 10 | 3 | 40 |
| 0.6 | 8 | 0.6 | 45 | 1.5 | 540 | 360 | 70 | 15 | 5 | 50 |
| 0.8 | 9 | 0.9 | 100 | 2.0 | 800 | 800 | 150 | 15 | 10 | 70 |
| 1.0 | 11 | 1.3 | 200 | 2.5 | 800 | 800 | 200 | 10 | 10 | 90 |
| 1.4 | 16 | 1.6 | 300 | 3.0 | 800 | 800 | 250 | 10 | 10 | 120 |
| 1.6 | 18 | 1.8 | 400 | 3.0 | 1200 | 1200 | 350 | 18 | 15 | 150 |
| 1.7 | 18 | 2.0 | 400 | 3.0 | 1200 | 1200 | 400 | 18 | 15 | 150 |
| 1.7 | 19 | 2.2 | 400 | 3.0 | 800 | 800 | 350 | 10 | 15 | 150 |
| 1.6 | 18 | 2.2 | 400 | 3.0 | 800 | 800 | 350 | 10 | 15 | 150 |
| 1.4 | 16 | 2.2 | 400 | 3.0 | 800 | 800 | 350 | 10 | 15 | 150 |
| 1.3 | 15 | 1.8 | 400 | 3.0 | 1200 | 1200 | 300 | 18 | 15 | 150 |
| 1.3 | 14 | 2.0 | 400 | 3.0 | 1200 | 1200 | 300 | 18 | 15 | 150 |
| 1.3 | 14 | 2.0 | 400 | 3.0 | 800 | 800 | 300 | 18 | 15 | 150 |
| 1.2 | 13 | 2.0 | 400 | 3.0 | 800 | 800 | 300 | 18 | 15 | 150 |
| 1.2 | 13 | 2.0 | 400 | 3.0 | 800 | 800 | 300 | 10 | 15 | 150 |
| +0.3 | +2 | +0.6 | +400 | +1.0 | +400 | +400 | +150 | h | +5 | +25 |
| +0.5 | +5 | +0.5 | +100 | +1.0 | +400 | +400 | +150 | h | +10 | +50 |

[f]The folacin allowances refer to dietary sources as determined by *Lactobacillus casei* assay after treatment with enzymes (conjugases) to make polyglutamyl forms of the vitamin available to the test organism.

[g]The recommended dietary allowance for vitamin B-$_{12}$ in infants is based on average concentration of the vitamin in human milk. The allowances after weaning are based on energy intake (as recommended by the American Academy of Pediatrics) and considerations of other factors, such as intestinal absorption.

[h]The increased requirement during pregnancy cannot be met by the iron content of habitual American diets nor by the existing iron stores of many women; therefore the use of 30-60 mg of supplemental iron is recommended. Iron needs during lactation are not substantially different from those of nonpregnant women, but continued supplementation of the mother for 2 to 3 months after parturition is advisable in order to replenish stores depleted by pregnancy.

standing the vast number of nutrients needed and the relative proportion of each required to maintain health is more important.

# NUTRITION: A CLOSER LOOK INSIDE

As you can see, eating is more than a pastime. The foods we eat are the source of the nutrients necessary for a healthy body. The

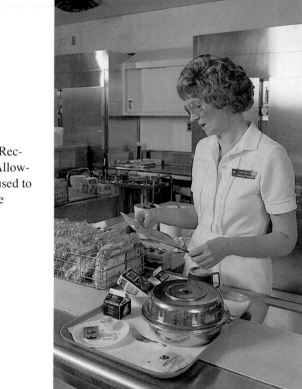

*Figure 1.9.* The Recommended Daily Allowances (RDAs) are used to plan meals for large groups of people.

science of nutrition provides us with a basis for understanding the function and source of the nutrients we need. Nutritionists, food scientists, biochemists, and doctors work together in nutrition research. Through this research, the scientific understanding of human nutrient needs continues to grow. Some nutrition questions still remain unanswered. However, we do have a body of scientific facts to guide us in making daily food choices.

How does the body change food to obtain nutrients for energy, bone formation, and muscle growth? What happens when we take in too little or too much of a nutrient? What factors shape your food habits? Answers to these questions, and many others, are discussed in the following chapters.

# CHECK YOUR PROGRESS

1. Define wellness.
2. Explain how knowing more about nutrition can be of value to you.
3. Define nutrient.
4. List the major classes of nutrients.
5. What is the most abundant nutrient in food?
6. List the three nutrients that provide energy.
7. Name the nutrient that is necessary for building body tissue.
8. Identify the organic nutrient needed in small amounts to regulate chemical reactions in the body.
9. Name the class of inorganic nutrients.
10. Do all people need the same nutrients? The same amounts? List factors affecting nutrient needs.
11. What are the Recommended Dietary Allowances (RDAs)? How do food and nutrition professionals use the RDAs?

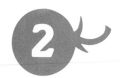 **YOUR NEED FOR ENERGY**

Maria complains of a headache and feels listless. Concentrating on her textbook seems impossible. Easily distracted, she gazes out the window at the autumn leaves blowing wildly in the wind. Suddenly, the gust of wind that had swirled the leaves frantically through the air stops. Energy, she thinks, is certainly a magical force. Wouldn't it be wonderful to be able to run like the wind? Today, just holding her book seems to take so much effort. Ever since she has been skipping meals to lose weight, Maria hasn't felt like doing much of anything.

Can what we eat really make a difference in the way we feel? As you will see, foods contain different nutrients. Each nutrient has a different function in the body. How do we obtain energy from the nutrients in food?

*In this chapter your objectives will be to:*

■ *Name different forms of energy*

■ *Identify the energy values of carbohydrates, fats, and proteins*

■ *Explain how the body changes food to obtain nutrients it needs*

■ *List the factors involved in determining human energy needs*

■ *Illustrate what is meant by energy balance*

## THE MAGIC OF ENERGY

*Energy* is defined as the capacity to do work. Energy, as a force, seems mysterious because it is invisible. We see or feel energy only when it is released to do work. There are many types of energy in nature, including *mechanical, electrical, nuclear,* and *chemical*. For

22

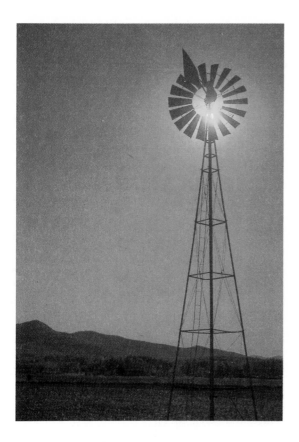

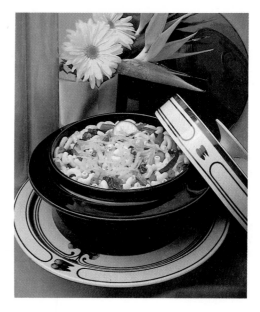

***Figure 2.1.***    Food is
one of many sources of
energy in nature.

example, the wind's energy can be caught by the long blades of a
windmill. The spinning blades transfer their energy of motion into
mechanical energy. This energy may be used to turn a belt that powers
an electric generator. The generator transforms the mechanical energy
into electrical current. When we flip the switch, the light bulb shines
brightly and gives off heat.

Food is a source of stored energy. The stored energy may be
converted by the body into electrical energy to conduct nerve impulses
or chemical energy to build body tissue. In addition, the stored energy
can be transferred into mechanical energy to power body muscles and
heat to maintain body temperature. Nutritionists have measured food
energy as heat. When food is *oxidized,* or burned, heat is released.
The amount of heat produced is measured in *kilocalories.* As
consumers we often say we are counting calories, when in fact we are

counting kilocalories (1000 calories = 1 kilocalorie). A *Calorie* (kilocalorie) is the amount of heat energy needed to raise the temperature of 1 kilogram of water 1° centigrade. In the metric system, the energy value of food would be described in *joules*; 1 kilocalorie equals 4.2 kilojoules.

Each nutrient has its own energy value based on a weight of 1 gram. Carbohydrate, the body's preferred fuel, provides 4 Calories per gram. Fat, the most concentrated energy source, provides 9 Calories per gram. Protein provides 4 Calories per gram, but is considered an expensive energy source. See Illustration 2.1. Recall that building body tissue is the major function of protein. When protein is burned for energy, it is lost as a building block. Where does the chemical energy in food come from?

## The Energy Cycle

The sun is the primary source of energy. Solar energy is captured by leaves in growing plants and converted to chemical energy in a process called *photosynthesis*. (See Illustration 2.2.) A green pigment, *chlorophyll,* present in leaves traps the sun's energy. Carbon dioxide from the air and water from the air and soil are drawn into the leaf. Carbon dioxide and water combine in the presence of solar energy to form glucose and oxygen.

*Glucose,* a sugar, is the simplest product of photosynthesis. The plant uses glucose to grow, develop roots, and produce fruit. The plant may store its energy as sugar, starch, or cellulose. A strawberry, for example, is a natural source of sugar, while a potato is mainly

*Illustration 2.1.*
Calories per Gram.

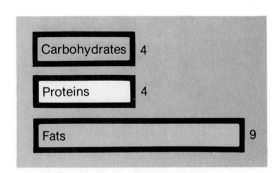

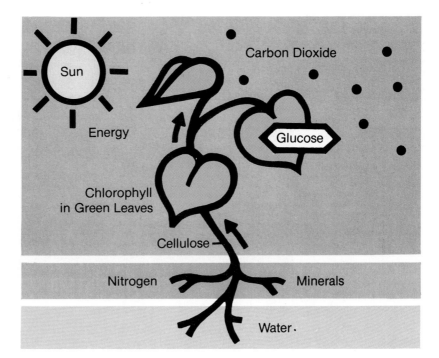

***Illustration 2.2.***
Photosynthesis.

starch. The stalk of celery is mainly cellulose. All three substances are known as *carbohydrates*.

The *oxygen* produced by the plant is released into the atmosphere for humans and animals to breathe. Indeed, the entire *food chain* begins with the amazing process of photosynthesis. In addition to capturing energy, plants are able to secure and use minerals and nitrogen from the soil. As a result, plants provide animals, fish, and humans with a food source that contains vitamins, minerals, protein, and energy. Many people choose to consume animal products as well as plants. The life-sustaining activities of animals (and humans) use oxygen and give off waste products, (including carbon dioxide, water, and nitrogen. These products return to the air and soil, from where plants absorb and use these elements to grow.

From their relationships in the food chain, we see how very dependent plants and animals are on one another. A change in number, distribution, or type of plants and animals (including people) can alter

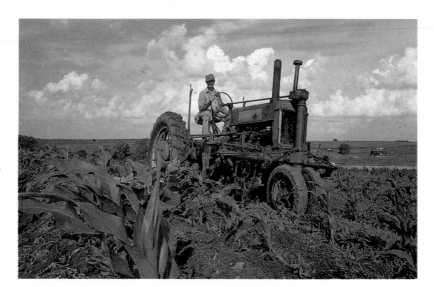

*Figure 2.2.* Photosynthesis is the first link in the food chain.

the natural balance of the food chain. This issue is a critical point in meeting the food demands of the world's rapidly growing human population.

## THE HUMAN MACHINE

The human body is a complex machine. Similar to a car, it needs an adequate fuel supply to operate. As mentioned in Chapter 1, the body's need for energy is second only to its requirement for water. Carbohydrates, fats, and proteins serve as the body's fuel supply. Running a marathon or swimming 50 laps requires a visible expenditure of energy. We may often forget, however, that energy is used by the body every second of every day for internal body processes. In fact, most of our energy is needed just to maintain body temperature.

Food as eaten is of little value to the body; it is the nutrients in the food we eat that the body requires. The body uses a highly involved process to break down and use food. The three steps of this process are digestion, absorption, and metabolism. The process also produces waste products, which are eliminated by means of excretion.

## Digestion

*Digestion* is a chemical and mechanical process for breaking down food. See Illustration 2.3. The process begins in the mouth with the mechanical action of chewing. At the same time, the *saliva* mixes with the food particles to split them apart in a process known as *hydrolysis*. Hydrolysis is aided by various *enzymes,* substances that speed up chemical reactions. Specific enzymes are needed to break apart carbohydrates, fats, and proteins. These enzymes do their work at different locations along the digestive tract.

The moist, small food particles are swallowed and moved down the esophagus into the stomach by the mechanical action of *peristalsis*. The mixture of food, water, and enzymes in the stomach is referred to as *chyme*. The chyme is further mixed with hydrochloric acid secreted by cells that line the stomach. Slowly the stomach contents are passed into the small intestine. A high-fat meal remains in the stomach longer than do foods containing starch or sugar. Thus fat provides *satiety,* or a feeling of fullness. Upon emptying into the intestine, the contents are *neutralized,* a process by which the acid is weakened. Final separation of food into the smallest nutrient units

*Figure 2.3.*
Whether resting or running, the human body uses energy every second of every day.

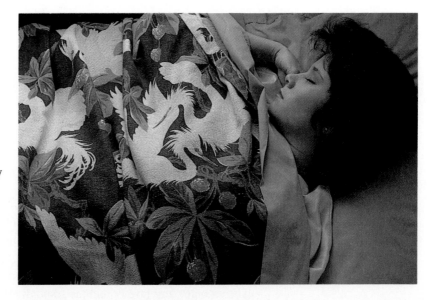

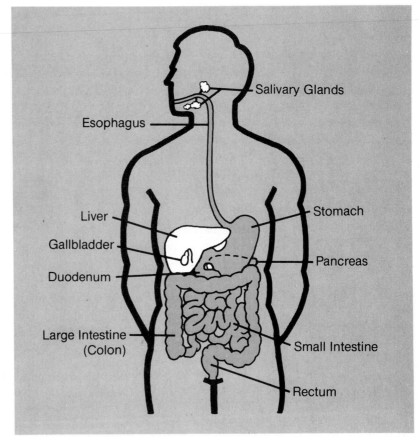

*Illustration 2.3.*
The Digestive System.

occurs in the small intestine. To illustrate, let's follow a hamburger and bun through the digestive process.

***Digestion of Carbohydrates.*** The hamburger bun is rich in the carbohydrate *starch*. Starch digestion begins in the mouth, where chewing the bun mechanically breaks it into smaller pieces. These pieces are coated with saliva, after which the enzyme *salivary amylase* begins to split the starch molecule chemically. The small moist particles of food are swallowed, moved down the esophagus, and enter the stomach.

The salivary amylase continues some digestive action until the acid environment of the stomach halts the process. After continued mixing with fluids, the chyme is released into the small intestine. The small intestine is the major site of carbohydrate digestion. The *pancreas* releases more amylase into the upper small intestine, further breaking down the starch. Cells lining the small intestine release enzymes to act on *maltose,* a sugar produced as a product of starch breakdown. *Maltase* splits the maltose into two glucose molecules. Glucose is the end product of starch, and one of the three sugars that enter the bloodstream. See Illustration 2.4. Now let's turn our attention to the hamburger.

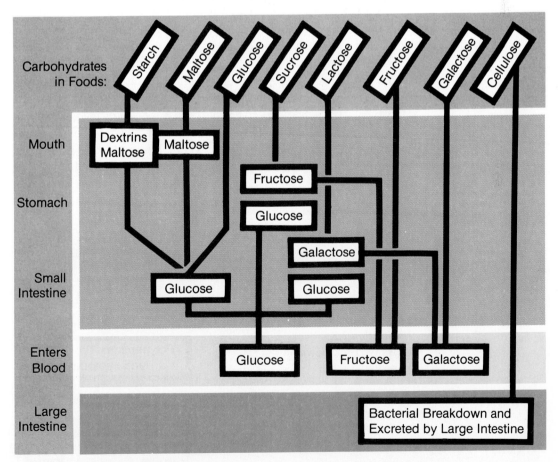

***Illustration 2.4.***   Digestive Breakdown of Carbohydrates.

***Digestion of Protein.*** The hamburger is a source of protein and fat. Let's first follow the digestion of protein. The meat is chewed and mixed with saliva in the mouth, then swallowed and moved down the esophagus to enter the stomach. Protein digestion begins in the stomach, where hydrochloric acid activates the enzyme *pepsin*. This enzyme splits the protein into simpler molecules, such as *polypeptides* (*poly-* means many), proteoses, and peptones. The chyme containing these smaller protein products is released into the small intestine and the enzyme *trypsin* is activated. Trypsin also activates additional protein enzymes. The simpler protein substances continue to be split apart, forming peptides and amino acids. *Amino acids* are the end products of protein digestion. See Illustration 2.5.

***Digestion of Fat.*** Fat digestion also begins in the stomach, with the action of the enzyme *gastric lipase*. This enzyme is able to break down short-chain *triglycerides* into their component (three) *fatty acids* and *glycerol*. (*Chain* length refers to the number of carbon atoms linked together.) Small- and medium-chain triglycerides can be then absorbed from the small intestine directly into the bloodstream. However, large-chain tryglycerides must be *emulsified,* or made soluble in water, before they can be broken down. These fats are released into the small intestine, where bile emulsifies the larger molecules. *Bile,* secreted by the liver, is stored in the gallbladder and

***Illustration 2.5.***
Digestive Breakdown of Proteins.

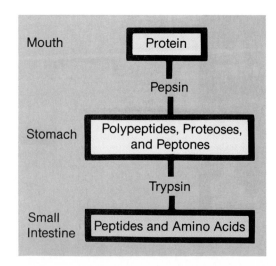

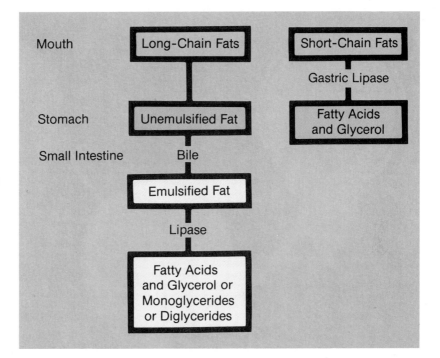

***Illustration 2.6.***
Digestive Breakdown
of Fats.

released into the small intestine when fat leaves the stomach. Bile emulsifies the fat globules, allowing them to mix with water-based digestive fluids. The pancreas releases the enzyme *lipase,* which splits the fat into the digestive end products of free fatty acids and glycerol. See Illustration 2.6.

## Absorption

When food has been separated into its simpler substances, the nutrients (including vitamins and minerals), can be absorbed from the small intestine into the bloodstream. The small intestine is about 21 feet long. The surface of the small intestine is specially designed to carry out the absorption process. The inner surface has hundreds of folds and projections called *villi.* See Illustration 2.7. The villi resemble hills and valleys on the interior of the intestine. On each villus are numerous surface projections called *microvilli,* which are only visible under a microscope. The villi and microvilli make almost

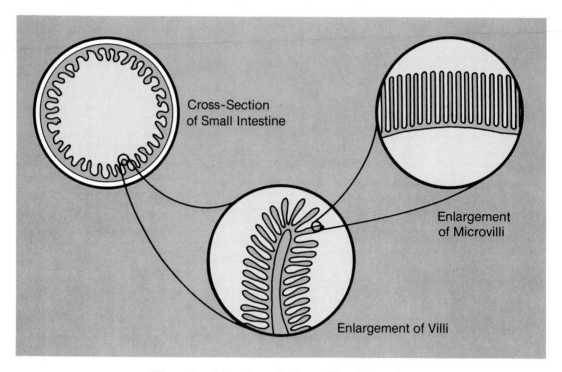

Cross-Section
of Small Intestine

Enlargement
of Microvilli

Enlargement of Villi

*Illustration 2.7.*     Inner Surface of Small Intestine.

600 times more surface area available for nutrients to cross the intestinal wall. Thus the area available for absorption is equal to half a basketball court.

The nutrient end products of digestion compete for space to be absorbed. The process of absorption may be accomplished by several means. Molecules may be passively diffused in a process called *osmosis.* Some molecules may be carried across the intestinal membrane with the help of another molecule. This process is referred to as *carrier-mediated diffusion.* See Illustration 2.8. When the concentration of molecules is greater in the bloodstream, energy must be expended to "pump" nutrients across the membrane. Some very large molecules require membrane cells to surround and swallow the molecule. This process is known as *pinocytosis.*

After crossing the intestinal membrane, the nutrient substances from carbohydrate and protein digestion travel through the *portal*

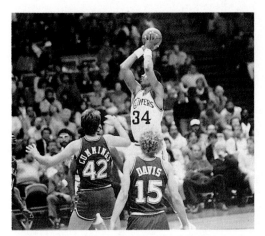

**Figure 2.4.** The area available for absorption in the small intestine is equal to half a basketball court.

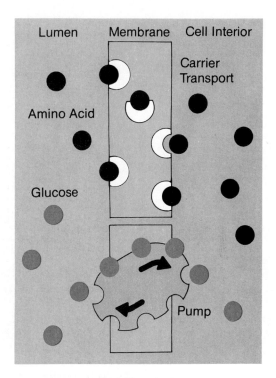

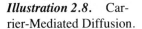

**Illustration 2.8.** Carrier-Mediated Diffusion.

*bloodstream* to various body tissues. Fat, however, takes a different route. The long-chain fatty acids are encased in a protein shell and travel initially through the *lymph system*. They finally enter the portal blood system through the *thoracic duct*. As noted earlier, small- and medium-chain fatty acids can be absorbed directly into the bloodstream from the stomach. See Illustration 2.9.

## Metabolism

*Metabolism,* the process of building up and breaking down body tissue, is the work of the *cell*. In the blood, energy nutrients are circulated to cells. Cells are the basic structural unit of the body. They are specialized with different tasks to accomplish. We have, for example, fat cells, nerve cells, and muscle cells. See Illustration 2.10.

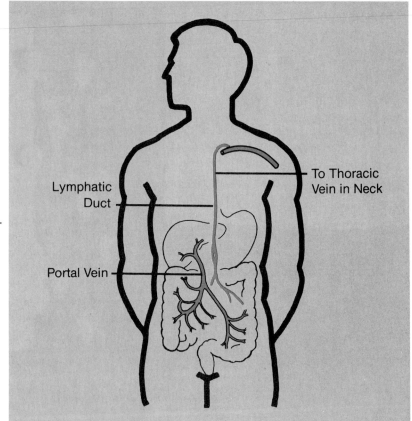

*Illustration 2.9.* Nutrient Transport System.

Each cell is responsible for changing the energy nutrient it needs into the fuel necessary to do its work. Cells require energy to build tissue, and energy is released when tissue is broken down.

Some nutrients may be stored, while others may be immediately used to provide energy for growth and activity. Each nutrient has a different capacity for storage and is pulled out of reserve in a set pattern as needed. The most readily available stored energy is *glycogen,* or the body's starch. Small amounts of glycogen are stored in muscle tissue and in the liver. When glycogen reserves are exhausted, *adipose tissue,* or fat, is broken down. Muscle tissue, or protein, may also be broken down to obtain energy. Obviously it is not desirable to break down muscle mass for energy.

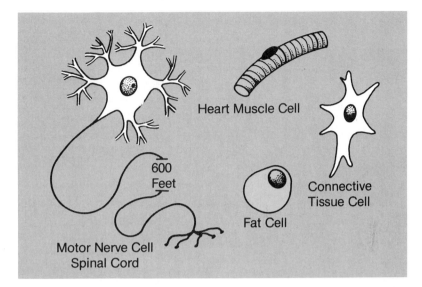

***Illustration 2.10.***
Various Types of Cells.

Cells specialize and unite to form body organs that carry out our internal activities. For example, the heart is composed of millions of cells working together to perform a specific function: to pump blood nonstop throughout the body. Energy is required for the lungs to expand and contract with each breath we take. The brain needs fuel to

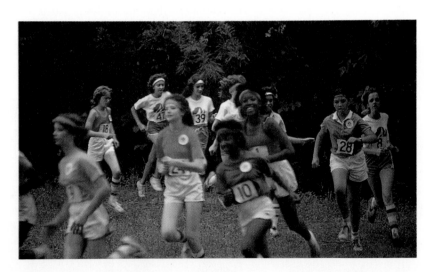

***Figure 2.5.*** Water and minerals may leave the body through perspiration from the skin.

process, sort, and direct our thoughts and actions. These and other internal activities all require energy.

## Excretion

Digestive and metabolic processes produce waste products that must be eliminated from the body. The kidneys filter out such metabolic wastes as urea and excess minerals. The large intestine is responsible for the excretion of undigested products, like fiber and bacteria. The lungs provide an avenue for exhaling another waste, carbon dioxide. Water and minerals may also leave the body through perspiration from the skin.

## Energy for Internal Operations

Energy is required for the body's internal operations, or *basal metabolism*. The rate at which energy is used for internal activities is known as the *basal metabolic rate* (BMR). The BMR is influenced by age, sex, body size, and health status. Infants and teenagers have the highest BMR, because extra energy is needed for growth. The elderly have the lowest value. An illness, especially if accompanied by a fever, raises the metabolic rate. Injury or surgery creates an extra demand for Calories to repair tissue.

Nutrition scientists have used various methods to determine how much energy a person expends. They can directly measure the oxygen consumed by the body or determine energy needs based on an individual's body surface area. A mathematical formula can be used to

### Table 2.1    Estimating Your Basal Metabolic Needs

18-year-old female weighing 125 pounds
125 pounds $\div$ 2.2 = 56.8 kilograms
56.8 $\times$ 22 = 1249 Calories

18-year-old male weighing 180 pounds
180 pounds $\div$ 2.2 = 81.8 kilograms
81.8 $\times$ 24 = 1963 Calories

quickly estimate basal energy needs. To calculate your basal needs, first change your body weight from pounds to kilograms by dividing pounds by 2.2. Then for a woman, multiply your weight in kilograms by 22. For a man, multiply your weight in kilograms by 24. Amazingly, between 1100 and 1800 Calories may be necessary to support your body's needs while at rest! See Table 2.1.

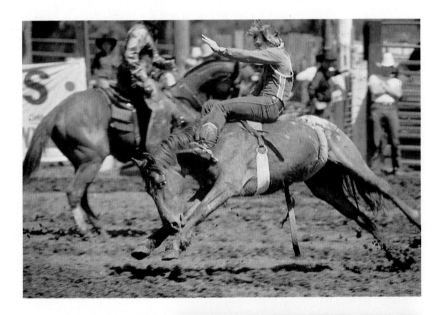

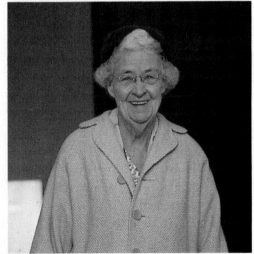

*Figure 2.6.* Individuals vary in the amount of Calories needed for daily activities.

## Go Power

In addition to BMR, people also vary in activity level. Thus the amount of fuel, or Calories, required for daily activities varies from person to person. A 6-foot tall male hockey player may need 3500 Calories, whereas a petite female executive may require only 1800 Calories. Even an individual's energy need may change from day to day. For example, playing tennis on the weekend would increase the caloric requirement for someone who usually sits at a desk for 6 to 8 hours per day. The pace and length of time spent at an activity determines the total Calories expended during the day. Table 2.2 shows the Calories used per minute for various activities. Would you describe yourself as sedentary, moderately active, or very active? One

### Table 2.2   Calories Expended for Various Activities*

| Activity | Cal/min | Activity | Cal/min |
|---|---|---|---|
| Sleeping | 1.2 | Dressing | 3.4 |
| Resting in bed | 1.3 | Showering | 3.4 |
| Sitting, normally | 1.3 | Driving motorcycle | 3.4 |
| Sitting, reading | 1.3 | Metal working | 3.5 |
| Lying, quietly | 1.3 | House painting | 3.5 |
| Sitting, eating | 1.5 | Cleaning windows | 3.7 |
| Sitting, playing cards | 1.5 | Carpentry | 3.8 |
| Standing, normally | 1.5 | Farming chores | 3.8 |
| Classwork, lecture (listen to) | 1.7 | Sweeping floors | 3.9 |
| Conversing | 1.8 | Plastering walls | 4.1 |
| Personal toilet | 2.0 | Truck and automobile repair | 4.2 |
| Sitting, writing | 2.6 | Ironing clothes | 4.2 |
| Standing, light activity | 2.6 | Farming, planting, hoeing, raking | 4.7 |
| Washing and dressing | 2.6 | Mixing cement | 4.7 |
| Washing and shaving | 2.6 | Mopping floors | 4.9 |
| Driving a car | 2.8 | Repaving roads | 5.0 |
| Washing clothes | 3.1 | Gardening, weeding | 5.6 |
| Walking indoors | 3.1 | Stacking lumber | 5.8 |
| Shining shoes | 3.2 | Chain saw | 6.2 |
| Making bed | 3.4 | | |

Source: B. J. Sharkey, *Physiology of Fitness* (Champaign, Ill.: Human Kinetics Publishers, 1979.) Used with permission.
*Depends on efficiency and body size. Add 10% for each 15 lb over 150, subtract 10% for each 15 lbs under 150.

## Table 2.2 (cont'd)

| Activity | Cal/min | Activity | Cal/min |
|---|---|---|---|
| Stone, masonry | 6.3 | Skipping rope | 10.0–15.0 |
| Pick-and-shovel work | 6.7 | Judo and karate | 13.0 |
| Farming, haying, plowing with | | Football (while active) | 13.3 |
|   horse | 6.7 | Wrestling | 14.4 |
| Shoveling (miners) | 6.8 | Skiing: | |
| Walking downstairs | 7.1 |   Moderate to Steep | 8.0–12.0 |
| Chopping wood | 7.5 |   Downhill Racing | 16.5 |
| Crosscut saw | 7.5–10.5 |   Cross-Country: 3–8 mph | 9.0–17.0 |
| Tree felling (ax) | 8.4–12.7 | Swimming: | |
| Gardening, digging | 8.6 |   Pleasure | 6.0 |
| Walking upstairs | 10.0–18.0 |   Crawl: 25–50 yd/min | 6.0–12.5 |
| Pool or billiards | 1.8 |   Butterfly: 50 yd/min | 14.0 |
| Canoeing: 2.5 mph– | |   Backstroke: 25–50 | |
|   4.0 mph | 3.0–7.0 |     yd/min | 6.0–12.5 |
| Volleyball: Recreational– | |   Breaststroke: 25–50 | |
|   Competitive | 3.5–8.0 |     yd/min | 6.0–12.5 |
| Golf: Foursome–Twosome | 3.7–5.0 |   Sidestroke: 40 yd/min | 11.0 |
| Horseshoes | 3.8 | Dancing: | |
| Baseball (except pitcher) | 4.7 |   Modern: Moderate– | |
| Ping Pong–Table Tennis | 4.9–7.0 |     Vigorous | 4.2–5.7 |
| Calisthenics | 5.0 |   Ballroom: Waltz– | |
| Rowing: Pleasure– | |     Rhumba | 5.7–7.0 |
|   Vigorous | 5.0–15.0 |   Square | 7.7 |
| Cycling: 5–15 mph (10 | | Walking: | |
|   speed) | 5.0–12.0 |   Road–Field (3.5 mph) | 5.6–7.0 |
| Skating: Recreation– | |   Snow: Hard–Soft | |
|   Vigorous | 5.0–15.0 |     (3.5–2.5 mph) | 10.0–20.0 |
| Archery | 5.2 |   Uphill: 5%–10%–15% | |
| Badminton: Recreational– | |     (3.5 mph) | 8.0–11.0–15.0 |
|   Competitive | 5.2–10.0 |   Downhill: 5%–10% | |
| Basketball: Half–Full Court | |     (2.5 mph) | 3.6–3.5 |
|   (more for fast break) | 6.0–9.0 |     15%–20% | |
| Bowling (while active) | 7.0 |     (2.5 mph) | 3.7–4.3 |
| Tennis: Recreational– | |   Hiking: 40 lb pack | |
|   Competitive | 7.0–11.0 |     (3.0 mph) | 6.8 |
| Water Skiing | 8.0 | Running: | |
| Soccer | 9.0 |   12 min mile (5 mph) | 10.0 |
| Snowshoeing (2.5 mph) | 9.0 |   8 min mile (7.5 mph) | 15.0 |
| Handball and squash | 10.0 |   6 min mile (10 mph) | 20.0 |
| Mountain climbing | 10.0 |   5 min mile (12 mph) | 25.0 |

method to determine energy needs for muscle activity is to keep a 24-hour activity record. A quick estimate can also be made by multiplying your basal energy level by 20% to 50%. To determine your energy output, use this formula:

1. Find your weight in kilograms

    ___?___ pounds ÷ 2.2 = ___?___ kilograms

2. Determine your basal energy needs
   a. Women

    ___?___ kilograms × 22 = ___?___ basal Calories
   b. Men

    ___?___ kilograms × 24 = ___?___ basal Calories

3. Estimate your energy needs for activity:

    Very Sedentary × 20% basal

    Sedentary × 30% basal

    Moderately Active × 40% basal

    Very Active × 50% basal

    ___?___ % × ___?___ basal Calories = ___?___ Calories for Activity

4. Calculate your SDE

    ___?___ basal Calories + ___?___ Calories for Activity = ___?___ Calories Expended

    ___?___ Calories Expended × 10% = ___?___ SDE Calories

5. Estimate of total energy output

    ___?___ basal Calories + ___?___ Calories for Activity + ___?___ SDE Calories = Total Calories Expended

Energy is also expended by the body to digest and absorb nutrients from food. The increased expenditure of energy to process food is known as *specific dynamic effect* (SDE). The energy used for this purpose ranges from 6% to 10% of the body's total energy expenditure. For example, if energy expended for basal metabolism and physical activity equals 2000 Calories, the SDE would be an extra 200 Calories (2000 × 10% = 200). Thus, total energy expended would be 2200 Calories. The SDE can also be determined based on actual Calories consumed.

## THE BALANCING GAME

Balancing total energy intake with output is one nutrition decision under your control. If your Calorie choices aren't matched by your needs, the body's internal control lets you know. Weight gain or loss is the visible result. Energy balance is achieved when Calorie intake equals energy output. When we feast, the body has a desire to save excess Calories for times of famine. Rarely do most of us encounter such limited intake, unless by choice. Taking in too few Calories means the body must pull stored energy out of reserves. The body stores only about 400 Calories of carbohydrate, so fat provides the major energy reserve. If other reserves are inadequate, the protein in muscle tissue may also be broken down for energy. As a result, it is important to know how many Calories you need to maintain your body weight. Use the formula given above to determine your energy need.

# FUELING THE HUMAN MACHINE

The human body has preferences as to the type of fuel required for certain tasks. Carbohydrates, fats, and proteins have unique roles in providing the body with energy. Chapter 3 discusses the body's use and storage of these energy nutrients. The· Chapter stresses food sources of carbohydrates, fats, and proteins and helps you evaluate your energy intake.

## CHECK YOUR PROGRESS

1. Give examples of several different forms of energy.
2. Identify the amount of energy provided by a gram of carbohydrate, fat, and protein.
3. How do plants get energy to grow? Describe the process of photosynthesis.
4. Describe the steps in the digestive process.
5. Where does nutrient absorption occur?
6. Define metabolism.
7. What is meant by basal metabolic rate (BMR)?
8. List four factors that influence basal metabolic rate. Who would have the higher BMR, a teenage girl or a 70-year-old woman? A man or a woman?
9. In addition to basal metabolism, what other factors determine the total amount of energy a person requires?
10. What is meant by energy balance?

# 3 ENERGY PLUS. . .

Sally said, "I can eat as much meat as I want to and not gain weight." Lisa asked, "But doesn't a hamburger have more Calories than a slice of bread?" "That doesn't matter, only starch makes you fat," replied Sally. Do you know who is right?

Freddie complained, "I never thought living on my own would be so much work. The hardest part is eating on a budget." "I know what you mean," said Jeff. "I need energy to play softball, but I can't afford to buy a lot of meat." What advice would you provide?

*In this chapter your objectives will be to:*

- *Describe how the body uses and stores the energy nutrients*
- *Identify food sources of carbohydrates, fats, and proteins*
- *Distinguish between low-fiber and high-fiber foods*
- *Identify food sources of saturated fat, unsaturated fat, and cholesterol*
- *Name examples of complete and incomplete proteins*
- *Calculate your caloric intake*

## THE CARBOHYDRATE CONNECTION

Whether we are reading a book or playing basketball, *carbohydrates* are the body's preferred fuel. Foods rich in carbohydrates are the most quickly digested and absorbed into the blood. How do carbohydrates in your diet provide you with quick energy?

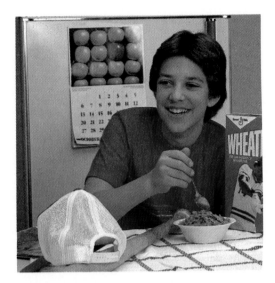

*Figure 3.1.*   Foods that
are rich in carbohydrates
are quickly digested and
absorbed for use as
energy.

## Sugar is Everywhere

Sugars are found in many natural and prepared foods. Most consumers associate the word sugar with the white, granulated substance they sprinkle on their cereal each morning. However, sugar is not just one substance. Sugars are the simplest form of carbohydrate. A variety of sugars exist in nature, each with a slightly different chemical structure. Thus they differ in taste, sweetness, and rate of metabolism. See Illustration 3.1.

Three simple sugars are glucose, fructose, and galactose. These sugars are known as *monosaccharides,* or single (*mono-* means one) sugars. *Glucose* is found in a variety of fruits and vegetables. In processed foods glucose is often listed on the label as corn syrup or dextrose. *Fructose,* also found in fruits and vegetables, is known as fruit sugar. Fructose is the sweetest of the sugars. *Galactose* is a major component of milk sugar.

When two single sugars are bonded together they form another simple sugar, a *disaccharide* (*di-* means two). Table sugar, or *sucrose,* for example, is composed of a unit of glucose and fructose. For use as table sugar, sucrose is obtained from sugar beets and sugar cane, but it is also present in maple syrup and molasses. Commercially, sucrose is added to many processed foods. Sucrose sweetens our beverages, candy, and breakfast cereals. To tempt our taste buds, cereals may be

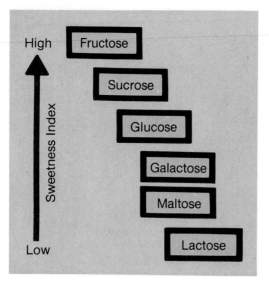

High

Fructose

Sucrose

Sweetness Index

Glucose

Galactose

Maltose

Lactose

Low

*Illustration 3.1.* The Relative Sweetness of Sugars.

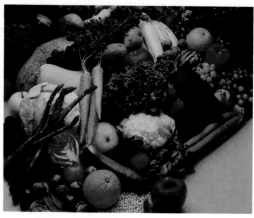

*Figure 3.2.* Glucose and fructose are two sugars commonly found in fruits and vegetables.

presweetened with both sucrose and high-fructose corn syrup. As you can see from Table 3.1, breakfast cereals vary greatly in their sugar content. In light of all the added sugar in our foods, it is little wonder that we Americans have developed a "sweet tooth."

*Lactose,* or milk sugar, is formed by joining galactose with glucose. Lactose is found in both human and cow's milk, but there is a greater quantity of it in cow's milk. This presents a problem for people who lack sufficient amounts of the enzyme *lactase.* A deficiency of this enzyme limits the body's ability to split lactose into galactose and glucose. As a result, persons with this deficiency cannot digest lactose and may suffer bloating, abdominal pain, and diarrhea after consuming milk. The problem may begin in infancy, childhood, or adulthood.

The reason for the enzyme deficiency is not completely understood, although the condition is more common among Blacks and Asians. One theory of its cause is related to how much milk your ancestors consumed. Drinking milk and eating milk products were common in Europe but not in most African and Asian countries. It is believed that the amount of lactase produced may be in proportion to the milk consumed. In other words, people over the years may biologically adapt to their food intake.

## Table 3.1    Sugar Content of Breakfast Cereals

| Product | Total Sugar[a] |
|---|---|
| Sugar Smacks (K) | 56.0% |
| Apple Jacks (K) | 54.6 |
| Froot Loops (K) | 48.0 |
| Sugar Corn Pops (K) | 46.0 |
| Super Sugar Crisp (GF) | 46.0 |
| Crazy Cow, chocolate (GM) | 45.6 |
| Corny Snaps (K) | 45.5 |
| Frosted Rice Krinkles (GF) | 44.0 |
| Frankenberry (GM) | 43.7 |
| Cookie Crisp, vanilla (R-P) | 43.5 |
| Cap'n Crunch, crunch berries (QO) | 43.3 |
| Cocoa Krispies (K) | 43.0 |
| Cocoa Pebbles (GF) | 42.6 |
| Fruity Pebbles (GF) | 42.5 |
| Lucky Charms (GM) | 42.2 |
| Cookie Crisp, chocolate (R-P) | 41.0 |
| Sugar Frosted Flakes of Corn (K) | 41.0 |
| Quisp (QO) | 40.7 |
| Crazy Cow, strawberry (GM) | 40.1 |
| Cookie Crisp, oatmeal (R-P) | 40.1 |
| Cap'n Crunch (QO) | 40.0 |
| Count Chocula (GM) | 39.5 |
| Alpha Bits (GF) | 38.0 |
| Honey Comb (GF) | 37.2 |
| Frosted Rice (K) | 37.0 |
| Trix (GM) | 35.9 |
| Cocoa Puffs (GM) | 33.3 |
| Cap'n Crunch, peanut butter (QO) | 32.2 |

*Continued*

Source: *Research News,* United States Department of Agriculture (Washington, D.C.: U.S. Government Printing Office, 1979).

Letters in parentheses after product name indicate manufacturers: General Foods (GF), General Mills (GM), Kellogg (K), Nabisco (N), Quaker Oats (QO), Ralston-Purina (R-P), Bio-Familia (BF), Organic Milling (OM), Pet (P).

[a]Sugar content is percent of dry weight and includes sucrose, glucose, fructose, maltose, and lactose.

[b]Granola-type cereal.

### Table 3.1 (cont'd)

| Product | Total Sugar[a] |
|---|---|
| Country Morning (K)[b] | 31.0 |
| Raisin Bran (GF) | 30.4 |
| Golden Grahams (GM) | 30.0 |
| Craklin' Bran (K) | 29.0 |
| Raisin Bran (K) | 29.0 |
| C.W. Post, Raisin (GF)[b] | 29.0 |
| Nature Valley Granola, Fruit and Nut (GM)[b] | 29.0 |
| C.W. Post (GF)[b] | 28.7 |
| Quaker 100% Natural, Raisin and Date (QO)[b] | 28.0 |
| Vita Crunch—Almond (OM)[b] | 28.0 |
| Vita Crunch—Raisin (OM)[b] | 27.0 |
| Heartland—Raisin (P)[b] | 26.0 |
| Frosted Mini Wheats (K) | 26.0 |
| Nature Valley Granola, Cinnamon and Raisin (GM)[b] | 25.0 |
| Quaker 100% Natural, Apple and Cinnamon (QO)[b] | 25.0 |
| Vita Crunch—Regular (OM)[b] | 24.0 |
| Familia (BF)[b] | 23.0 |
| Heartland, Coconut (P)[b] | 22.0 |
| Quaker 100% Natural, Brown Sugar & Honey (QO)[b] | 22.0 |
| Country Crisp (GF) | 22.0 |
| Life, cinnamon (QO) | 21.0 |
| 100% Bran (N) | 21.0 |
| All Bran (K) | 19.0 |
| Fortified Oat Flakes (GF) | 18.5 |
| Life (QO) | 16.0 |
| Team (N) | 14.1 |
| Grape Nuts Flakes (GF) | 13.3 |
| 40% Bran (GF) | 13.0 |
| Buckwheat (GM) | 12.2 |
| Product 19 (K) | 9.9 |
| Concentrate (K) | 9.3 |
| Total (GM) | 8.3 |

**Table 3.1 (cont'd)**

| Product | Total Sugar[a] |
|---|---|
| Wheaties (GM) | 8.2 |
| Rice Krispies (K) | 7.8 |
| Grape Nuts (GF) | 7.0 |
| Special K (K) | 5.4 |
| Corn Flakes (K) | 5.3 |
| Post Toasties (GF) | 5.0 |
| Kix (GM) | 4.8 |
| Rice Chex (R-P) | 4.4 |
| Corn Chex (R-P) | 4.0 |
| Wheat Chex (R-P) | 3.5 |
| Cheerios (GM) | 3.0 |
| Shredded Wheat (N) | 0.6 |
| Puffed Wheat (QO) | 0.5 |
| Puffed Rice (QO) | 0.1 |

Some people are able to consume small amounts of fluid milk if the enzyme deficiency is not severe. Other people may consume milk in other forms such as cheese and yogurt without any problems. Because milk is an important carrier of nutrients, a product was developed to allow people affected by lactase deficiency to drink milk. The commercial enzyme, LactAid, is added to fluid milk and breaks down most of the lactose before the milk is consumed. Commercial lactose-free nutritional formulas are also available for infants and adults.

Another sugar adds unique flavor to a chocolate malt. The sugar *maltose* is composed of two units of glucose linked together. It is found in cereal grains and fermented alcoholic beverages.

**Starch: The Complex Carbohydrate**

Starch is a *polysaccharide,* meaning it is composed of many sugars (*poly-* means many)—sometimes several hundreds. The arrangement of the units of glucose varies for each type of starch. Foods composed primarily of starch are potatoes, rice, wheat, corn, and

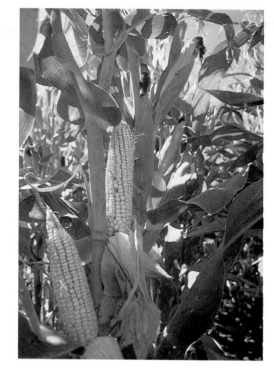

*Figure 3.3.* Corn, potatoes, rice, wheat, and legumes are prime sources of starch.

legumes. Winter squash and pumpkin are also high in starch content.

Starch is available in natural and refined forms in the foods we eat. Whole wheat bread, for example, contains the crushed, whole kernel of wheat. The kernel consists of an outer layer of *bran,* which contains nondigestible fiber and B vitamins. The whole kernel also contains a nutrient-rich portion called *germ.* The germ is an excellent source of vitamin E and the B vitamins niacin and riboflavin. It is the inner portion of the kernel, or *endosperm,* that is primarily starch. See Illustration 3.2.

Processed foods, such as white bread, are *refined,* meaning the bran layer and usually the germ have been removed. Thus processing also removes important nutrients. In some processed foods nutrients such as thiamin, riboflavin, and niacin are replaced. When nutrients are replaced to their natural levels the product is referred to as *enriched.* When extra amounts of a nutrient or other nutrients not originally in the food are added, the food is labeled *fortified.*

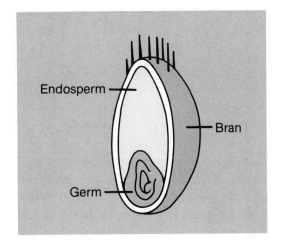

*Illustration 3.2.*  The
Wheat Kernel.

Complex carbohydrates in their natural forms are excellent sources of fiber. *Cellulose* is the main dietary fiber. Although cellulose cannot be broken down by the body for use as energy, it is important in keeping the digestive tract working smoothly. The typical American diet of highly processed foods is low in fiber. For many people constipation and diseases of the lower intestine are aggravating problems. Eating high-fiber foods is part of the recommended treatment for constipation. Consuming a diet higher in fiber may also help to prevent diseases of the colon, or lower intestine. High-fiber foods include whole grain products, bran, seeds, nuts, raw fruits, and raw vegetables. See Table 3.2. Refined, highly processed cereals, white bread, white rice, milk, and meats are low in fiber.

## Quick Energy

To be of use in providing energy, carbohydrates must be available in the body as single sugars. Complex carbohydrates must be broken down by digestion (refer to Chapter 2) before they are ready to be used. The amount of ready energy in the body is determined by measuring the blood glucose level. This level varies with the type, amount, and frequency of food consumed. For example, foods containing simple sugars and starch cause the level of blood glucose to rise rapidly. On the other hand, a mixture of carbohydrates, fats, and

**Table 3.2   Food Sources of Fiber**

| Food | Serving Size | Grams of Fiber | Food | Serving Size | Grams of Fiber |
|---|---|---|---|---|---|
| High-fiber and Bran Cereals | ½ cup | up to 13.5 | Brussels Spouts | 4 | 2.5 |
| Baked Beans | ½ cup | 8.3 | Peanut Butter | 2 tablespoons | 2.4 |
| Apple | 1 medium | 4.5 | Whole Wheat Bread | 1 slice | 1.8 |
| Broccoli, cooked | 1 med. stalk | 7.4 | Apricots | 3 medium | 2.3 |
| Coconut, shredded | 2"x2"x½" piece | 6.1 | Carrots, raw | 1 medium | 2.3 |
| Spinach, cooked | ½ cup | 5.7 | Beets | ½ cup | 2.1 |
| Blackberries | ½ cup | 5.3 | Peaches | 1 medium | 2.1 |
| Almonds | ¼ cup | 5.1 | Zucchini, raw | ½ cup | 2.0 |
| Kidney beans | ½ cup | 4.5 | String beans, raw | ½ cup | 2.0 |
| Cabbage, boiled, shredded | ½ cup | 2.0 | Puffed Wheat | 1 cup | 2.2 |
| Peas, cooked | ½ cup | 4.2 | Tomato, raw | 1 medium | 1.8 |
| White beans | ½ cup | 4.2 | Barley, raw | ½ cup | 1.8 |
| Banana | 1 medium | 4.0 | Miller's Bran | 1 tablespoon | 4.0 |
| Corn | ½ cup | 3.9 | Shredded Wheat | 1 biscuit | 3.1 |
| Potato | 1 medium | 3.9 | Onions, cooked | ½ cup | 1.6 |
| Pear | 1 medium | 3.8 | Strawberries | ½ cup | 1.6 |
| Lentils | ½ cup | 3.7 | Walnuts, chopped | ¼ cup | 1.6 |
| Lima beans, cooked | ½ cup | 3.5 | Asparagus, chopped | ½ cup | 1.2 |
| Sweet potato | 1 medium | 3.5 | Cherries | 10 | .8 |
| Pinto beans | ½ cup | 3.1 | Cauliflower, raw | ½ cup | 1.0 |
| Peanuts, chopped | ¼ cup | 2.9 | Pineapple | 3½"x¾" piece | 1.0 |
| Brown rice, raw | ½ cup | 2.8 | Asparagus | 4 med. spears | .9 |
| Cornflakes | 1 cup | 2.8 | White Bread | 1 slice | .8 |
| Orange | 1 medium | 2.6 | Celery, raw | 1 stalk | .7 |
| Raisins | ¼ cup | 2.5 | Onions, raw, chopped | ¼ cup | .6 |
|  |  |  | Plums | 3 medium | 1.8 |

Source: American Institute for Cancer Research, Dietary Fiber to Lower Cancer Risk. Reprinted with permission from the American Institute for Cancer Research (Washington, D.C.).

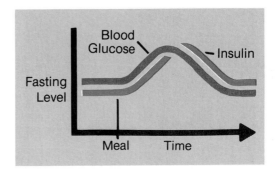

*Illustration 3.3.* Normal Blood Glucose—Insulin Response.

proteins, and the longer time it takes to break them down, result in more even blood glucose levels.

Protein substances known as *hormones* also control the blood glucose level. The hormone *insulin* is released by the pancreas to help cells draw in the available glucose for use as energy. When the amount of glucose available exceeds the cells' energy needs, insulin also acts to permit its storage either as *glycogen,* the body's starch, or as fat. The action of insulin lowers the level of glucose in the blood. See Illustration 3.3. *Diabetes mellitus* is a disorder in which the hormonal regulation of blood glucose is disrupted. Diabetes will be further explained in Chapter 6.

## Sugar Facts and Fiction

Popular food magazines and diet books have raised public awareness of the dangers of sugar overload. Unfortunately, not all you may have read is scientifically true. What do we know about the problems that result from eating excessive amounts of sugar?

The main health problem related to frequent intake of high-sugar foods is *tooth decay.* Sugary foods, particularly those of a sticky consistency, coat the teeth. The more often teeth are coated with sugar, the more opportunities bacteria have to break down the sugar. The acid formed from this bacterial action erodes tooth enamel, producing decay. See Illustration 3.4.

Obesity is also a major health problem in the United States. *Empty-calorie foods* are foods that lack other nutrients, and consuming many such products may contribute to excess Calorie intake. In

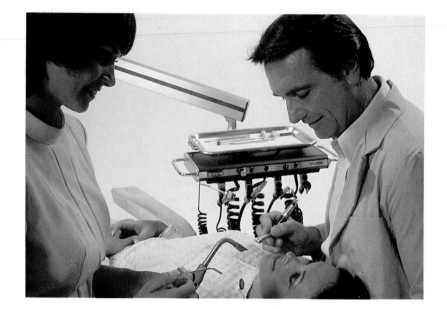

*Figure 3.4.*   Tooth decay is a serious problem related to eating foods high in sugar.

addition, these foods may replace other foods, such as whole grains and cereals, that contain needed nutrients. However, overconsumption of any food may lead to excess Calorie intake, and thus cause weight gain. Remember, you can gain weight by eating too much protein, fat, or carbohydrate.

*Illustration 3.4.*   Process of Tooth Decay.

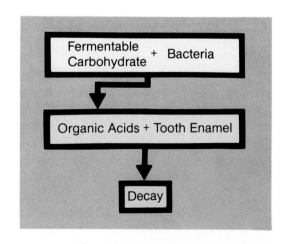

Low blood sugar levels, with accompanying signs of "sugar blues," have been blamed on eating too many sweets. Although some people do react to foods eaten, including sugar, feelings of depression and exhaustion cannot be blamed on sugar. Likewise, a relationship between sugar and hyperactivity has not been proven. Signs of hunger, sweating, and light-headedness may be reactions to food intake. However, diagnosed cases of low blood sugar levels caused by overeating sugars and sweets are very few.

## CONCENTRATED ENERGY

Contrary to popular belief, bread and potatoes are not the Calorie culprits dieters need fear. Bread and potatoes are carbohydrate foods that supply 4 Calories per gram. In other words, a slice of bread contains 65 Calories, whereas a baked potato supplies 145 Calories. However, it is the butter, margarine, or sour cream that is added that sends the Calorie values soaring. Fats provide the most concentrated source of energy, 9 Calories per gram. This translates into 35 Calories for a teaspoon of butter or margarine. A tablespoon of sour cream adds 25 Calories. Thus while fats add flavor, they also add extra Calories.

Dietary fat is one of the most controversial issues in nutrition today. How much fat do we need? Are all dietary fats alike?

*Figure 3.5.* Potatoes are low in calories—until they are topped with butter and sour cream.

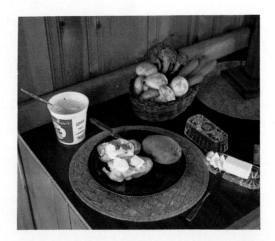

## Americans Love the Taste

Fats such as butter and salad dressing are visible parts of our meals. A person is usually aware of adding these fats to other foods. However, other sources of fat that we may not think about include fried foods, meats, and many dairy products. Obviously, the total fat consumed each day dramatically affects caloric intake.

A small amount of fat in the diet is necessary. In addition to providing energy, dietary fat is a carrier of the fat-soluble vitamins A, D, E, and K. It is also essential for the body to obtain one fatty acid, *linoleic acid,* from food sources.

Fat is also a component of cell membranes. When stored as fat tissue, it serves as an insulator in maintaining body temperature. Fat also protects internal body organs. Men and women differ in their body composition. Between 14% and 16% of the body weight of men is fat. In women, fat represents about 20% to 23% of body weight. These higher fat reserves prepare a woman's body to meet the energy demands of pregnancy.

The percentage of body fat may be altered by exercise and severe weight loss. For example, a marathon runner's body fat content

*Figure 3.6.* Exercise can alter a person's percentage of body fat.

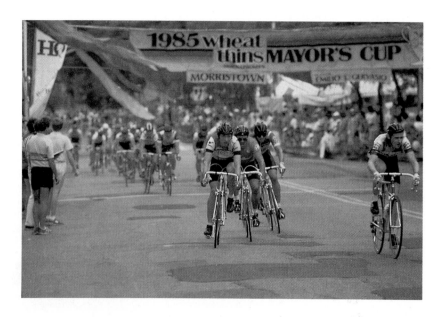

may be as low as 5%. Menstruation may be interrupted or halted in women with very low fat stores. This unnatural condition often occurs in gravely ill or starving persons.

The amount of fat people should consume each day is debatable. A deficiency of fat is highly unlikely in the American population. In the typical American diet, fat may provide as much as 42% of the total Calories. This high-fat intake has been linked with the incidence of heart disease and breast and colon cancer. However, the type of fat consumed may be just as important as the total amount.

## Fat: There is a Difference

Most dietary fat is composed of triglycerides. Each *triglyceride* is formed from three fatty acids and glycerol. However, not all fatty acids are alike. Fatty acids have carbon *chains,* or links, that may be short, medium, or long. Short- and medium-chain fatty acids, with less than 12 carbon atoms, are more easily absorbed. Perhaps of more importance is that fatty acids may be saturated or unsaturated. The carbon atoms of a *saturated fatty acid* have all the hydrogen atoms they can accept, whereas an *unsaturated fatty acid* is still able to accept more hydrogen atoms. The degree of saturation is independent of the length of the carbon chain.

A diet high in saturated fats tends to raise blood cholesterol levels. On the other hand, consuming polyunsaturated and monosaturated fats appears to lower blood cholesterol levels. This topic is discussed in Chapter 6.

Animal products, such as milk, butter, and meat, are higher in saturated fat content. Vegetable oils, such as corn and soy oil, contain primarily unsaturated fatty acids. The exceptions are palm and coconut oils which are highly saturated. These are commonly used in commercial whipped toppings, coffee whiteners, and other processed foods. See Table 3.3.

Saturated fats are usually solid at room temperature, whereas polyunsaturated fats are liquid. *Food technologists,* scientists who develop new food products, use a process called *hydrogenation* to chemically add hydrogen to oils. The more hydrogen added, the more solid the product becomes. This process is used to make shortening and margarine. This process also makes the product more saturated than its oil in natural form. Recall how refining and processing

## Table 3.3    Common Saturated and Unsaturated Fats

### Saturated Fats

| | | |
|---|---|---|
| Beef | Coconut Oil | Palm Oil |
| Butter | Cream | Pork |
| Cheese | Lard | Veal |
| Chicken | Milk | |
| Chocolate | Palm Kernel Oil | |

### Unsaturated Fats

*Monounsaturated Fats*

| | | |
|---|---|---|
| Almonds | Flounder | Olive Oil |
| Avocados | Haddock | Peanut Oil |
| Cottonseed Oil | Margarine | Peanuts |

*Polyunsaturated Fats*

| | | |
|---|---|---|
| Corn Oil | Sesame Oil | Sunflower Oil |
| Mayonnaise | Soft Margarine | |
| Safflower Oil | Soybean Oil | |

Source: *American Institute for Cancer Research Newsletter.* Reprinted with permission from the American Institute for Cancer Research (Washington, D.C.: Spring 1985).

changed the whole wheat kernel. In a similar manner, fats and oils can be changed by processing.

Oxygen causes oil to break down. Thus when exposed to heat and air, oil becomes rancid, or spoils. Hydrogenation decreases spoilage. During processing of oils the preservatives BHA (butylated hydroxyanisole) and BHT (butylated hydroxytoluene) may also be added to prevent spoilage. These substances are called *antioxidants* because they limit oxygen's breakdown of fat.

Did you know that a tablespoon of margarine and butter both contain 100 Calories? By law they must contain 80% fat. However, diet margarines may have more water added. Whipped butter has air incorporated into it. Thus both have fewer Calories per tablespoon than margarine or butter.

***Figure 3.7.*** Hydrogenation is a process
whereby hydrogen is
chemically added to oils
to make them more
solid.

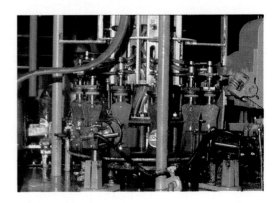

## Cholesterol: An Animal Product

Another fatlike substance that is important in several body
processes is *cholesterol.* It is made by the body and is also available in
foods. However, only foods of animal origin contain cholesterol.
Organ meats, such as liver and egg yolk, are the highest sources.

## Table 3.4    Cholesterol Content of Selected Foods

| Food Item | Amount | Cholesterol (mg) |
|---|---|---|
| Liver (beef, pork) | 3 oz slice | 372 |
| Egg Yolk | 1 large | 252 |
| Shrimp, canned | ½ cup | 96 |
| Crab, canned | ½ cup | 80 |
| Beef | 3 oz | 80 |
| Halibut | 1 fillet | 75 |
| Chicken, breast | ½ breast | 63 |
| Lobster | ½ cup meat | 61 |
| Oysters, canned | 3 oz | 38 |
| Milk, Whole | 1 cup | 34 |
| Cheese, Cheddar | 1 oz | 28 |
| Ice Cream | ½ cup | 26 |
| Cheese, Cottage, 1% fat | 1 cup | 23 |

Source: Adapted from R. M. Feeley, P. E. Criner, and B. K. Watt, Cholesterol content of foods, *Journal of the American Dietetic Association,* 1972, vol. 61, p. 134.

Other foods that contain cholesterol include seafood, beef, pork, chicken, milk, cheese, and butter. See Table 3.4. The effect of a high blood cholesterol level on the development of heart and circulatory diseases will be discussed in Chapter 6.

# PROTEIN FOR GROWTH AND REPAIR

Advertisements often promote the wonders of protein. Commercials for protein-enriched shampoos claim to heal the damaged, split ends of hair. Amazing results are promised with liquid protein weight loss diets. Protein-rich health drinks are featured as a must for muscle-building athletes. Gelatin, a protein, has been the traditional remedy for weak, chipped fingernails. Can protein really work these cosmetic wonders? To judge the validity of these claims, it is necessary to know more about protein.

The name protein comes from a Greek word meaning "of first importance." Indeed, protein serves a more important, specialized role than providing energy. Proteins are substances that make life itself possible. All living organisms contain protein. What makes protein so special?

## Building Proteins

Like carbohydrates and fats, proteins also contain carbon, hydrogen, and oxygen. In addition, they contain nitrogen. This nitrogen is packaged in units called *amino acids*. There are 22 different amino acids. Amino acids join together to build proteins, much like we use letters of the alphabet to form words. There are endless combinations, with most proteins containing several hundred amino acids.

The number and arrangement of amino acids determine what the protein will be. Protein in wheat is different than that in corn, and both are different than that in beef. Your body also produces many different proteins. To do so, the body needs a ready supply of amino acids. Many amino acids can be made by the body, but eight essential ones cannot. In nutrition, *essential nutrient* means a nutrient that cannot be made by the body. Thus it must be obtained from food sources. See Table 3.5.

**Table 3.5    Essential Amino Acids**

Isoleucine
Leucine
Lysine
Methionine
Phenylalanine
Threonine
Tryptophan
Valine

## Complete and Incomplete Proteins

Not all foods are equal sources of the eight essential amino acids. Animal products, such as meat, milk, and eggs, contain an amount of these eight adequate to support human growth. These foods are considered to be complete proteins. Plant proteins, like corn, wheat, peanuts, and dried beans, are low in one or more of the essential amino acids. Thus they are labeled incomplete proteins. See Table 3.6. When eaten with another food containing the missing amino acid, the mixture is then complete. Foods that enhance the protein quality of another food are described as *complementary proteins*. This process of protein supplementation will be described in detail in Chapter 13.

**Table 3.6    Proteins in Common Foods**

| Complete Proteins | Incomplete Proteins |
|---|---|
| Milk | Dried beans and peas |
| Meat | Grains |
| Fish | Seeds and Nuts |
| Cheese | |
| Eggs | |
| Poultry | |

## Protein: Its Many Roles

***Tissue growth and repair.*** The body uses amino acids to produce a variety of proteins, each of which has a special purpose. Body tissue, such as muscle, skin, hair, and nails, contain protein. In a growing child there is a constant demand for new body tissue. Thus a growing child's need for protein is proportionately higher. For everyone there is an ongoing need to repair worn-out cells. Some cells need to be replaced more often than others. For example, cells lining your intestinal tract completely *turn over,* or replace themselves, every 4 days. Alternatively, the turnover of all your skin cells may take a number of years. See Table 3.7 to identify the amount of protein you require in your diet each day.

Tissue is formed from the inside out. Therefore, protein applied to the surface of hair or skin will not be absorbed into the tissue. Protein shampoos, for example, only temporarily coat the split hair shaft.

***Enzymes.*** Enzymes, the substances that enable chemical reactions to occur, also contain protein. There are thousands of

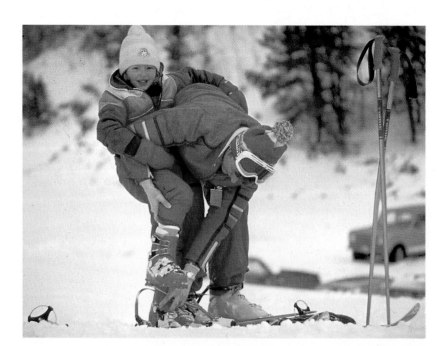

*Figure 3.8.* A growing child requires adequate protein to build new body tissue.

## Table 3.7    Required Amount of Protein per Day

| Age (yr) | Daily Total (gm) |
|---|---|
| Males | |
| 11-14............... | 45 |
| 15-18............... | 56 |
| 19-22............... | 56 |
| Females | |
| 11-14............... | 46 |
| 15-18............... | 46 |
| 19-22............... | 44 |

Source: Food and Nutrition Board, National Academy of Science, National Research Council, *Recommended Dietary Allowances,* ed. 9 (Washington, D.C.: National Academy Press, 1980); (available from Office of Publications, National Academy of Sciences, 2101 Constitution Ave., N.W., Washington, D.C. 20418).

enzymes in each cell. Each enzyme helps form or separate compounds the body needs.

*Proteins in the Blood.* Protein plays a role in the body's water balance. *Albumin* holds water within the blood vessel. A decrease in the albumin level may cause fluid to escape into tissue. The result is *edema,* a swelling produced by the accumulating fluid. Have you noticed in photographs the swollen bellies of poorly nourished African children? This is severe edema caused by a lack of protein.

Another protein that is found in red blood cells is *hemoglobin.* This iron-containing protein complex carries oxygen from the lungs to all body tissues. It also carries carbon dioxide, a waste product, back to the lungs to be exhaled.

*Buffers.* Proteins also act as buffers to regulate the *pH,* or acidity of the blood. You can think of pH as a sliding scale from 1 to 14, with 1 the most acidic and 14 the most basic. The normal pH of blood is 7.35 to 7.45, or slightly basic. As buffers, proteins have the ability to form acids or bases to keep the blood pH in a safe range. A protein will become acidic or basic depending on what the body needs to maintain normal pH.

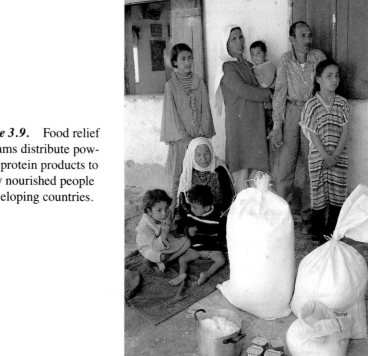

***Figure 3.9.***    Food relief
programs distribute pow-
dered protein products to
poorly nourished people
in developing countries.

***Hormones and Antibodies.*** Some hormones are made of
proteins. An example discussed earlier is *insulin,* which regulates the
blood glucose level.

The body's defense system is composed of proteins known as
*antibodies.* Antibodies are formed in response to invading particles.
Bacteria, viruses, and even foods may provoke the body to produce
antibodies. The body's ability to produce adequate antibodies provides
an *immunity,* or protection from the invader. This is the principle
behind vaccinations for such diseases as polio and measles. Antibody
formation is a sensitive measure of the body's protein status.

***Protein for Energy: The Last Resort.*** Finally, protein may
also be used for energy if the supply of fats and carbohydrates is
inadequate. Energy demands take top priority. When protein is used
for energy, it is lost for use in its many other roles. The nitrogen from

the amino acids is split off and excreted as urea. This is why it is expensive to your body to follow a high-protein, low-carbohydrate diet. The protein consumed may be sacrificed for energy needs. In addition, your kidneys will be working very hard to flush out the unused nitrogen. Any diet of this type requires a daily fluid intake of 8 to 10 glasses of water or other liquid. The weight lost in this diet is because of a decrease in total Calories consumed and the slight increase in energy required to metabolize protein.

**Table 3.8    Determining Your Caloric Intake**

| Foods Eaten | Quantity Eaten | Calories per Standard Serving | Calories for Size Portion Eaten |
|---|---|---|---|
| | | | |
| | | | |
| | | | |
| | | | |

**Total Calories Consumed:**

## HOW MANY CALORIES DO YOU CONSUME?

For many years food scientists have analyzed the content of foods to determine their caloric and nutrient value. Results of their research have been compiled into food composition tables. Two of the most widely used tables are the United States Department of Agriculture Handbook No. 456 and the Home and Garden Bulletin No. 72. The latter bulletin is included as a reference in the Appendix of this text.

To determine your typical caloric intake, record the foods eaten during 1 day on a form similar to Table 3.8. Next, identify the caloric content of each food item by locating the food, its method of preparation, and nearest portion size in the Appendix food composition table. Record the caloric value listed. Adjust the value to reflect the amount eaten. For example, if the given portion is ½ cup and you consumed 1 cup, simply multiply the Calorie figure by 2. Record the caloric value of each food eaten during that day. Finally, add the caloric values together to obtain your total energy intake.

If you have access to a computer, this task may be less time consuming. Today many computer diet analysis programs are available. These software packages use various food composition tables to build their data base. When you enter the data for a food item and

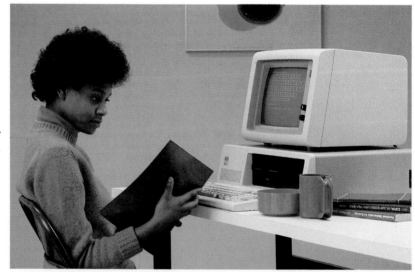

*Figure 3.10.* Diet analysis is made easier with the use of specially designed computer software.

portion size, the computer searches out the caloric value and/or nutrient content. Computer programs may provide you with a detailed assessment of your diet. Some programs will even offer hints for improving your diet.

Compare your caloric intake with the individual energy needs described in Chapter 2. If these figures are similar, the quantity of food you are eating is appropriate to meet your needs. In other words, you are in *energy balance*. If not, do you find yourself gaining or losing weight? Tips for achieving and maintaining your desirable weight are covered in Chapter 7.

The amount of food energy you consume isn't your only nutritional concern. The nutritional quality of the foods you eat is as important as the quantity. Just as foods differ in caloric value, they also vary in vitamin and mineral content. Read on to see what you may be missing!

## CHECK YOUR PROGRESS

1. What is the major function of a carbohydrate? Describe its simplest form.
2. Define monosaccharide, disaccharide, and polysaccaride. Give an example and food source of each.
3. What is fiber? Give an example of a high-fiber food. Explain the value of eating foods high in fiber.
4. Name the major health problem related to eating too much sugar.
5. In which form is most dietary fat? Name the two chemical substances that combine to make this fat.
6. Define saturated and unsaturated fat. Give a food example of each.
7. Name the vegetable oils that are saturated fats.
8. Define hydrogenation. Give an example of a product that is hydrogenated.
9. Explain the purpose of an antioxidant. Give an example of an antioxidant.
10. Which of these foods are sources of cholesterol? Butter, corn oil, coconut oil, egg yolk, meat, peanuts.
11. Identify several functions protein has in the body?

12. Name the basic building blocks of protein.
13. What is meant by essential? How many amino acids are considered essential for the adult?
14. How do complete and incomplete protein differ? Name three foods that are complete proteins and three foods that are incomplete proteins.

# THE REGULATORS

"I don't have time for breakfast, so I take a vitamin pill every day," exclaimed Carl.

"I always have time for cereal," replied Sara. "One bowl of fortified cereal gives me 100% of the vitamins I need each day."

Sam declared, "I only eat natural foods, like granola, for breakfast. Natural vitamins are the best."

"Minerals are important, too. Don't women need more iron than men?" asked Annette.

Is taking a vitamin pill a substitute for not eating right? In search of better health, Americans spend millions of dollars each year on megavitamin supplements. Less publicized, but perhaps as confusing to consumers, are the minerals. Obtaining enough of some minerals is a concern, but too much of other minerals may also be a problem. As you will see, foods are not equal in their vitamin and mineral content. Gathering a few vitamin and mineral facts will enable you to add nutritional quality to your diet. Let this knowledge be your guide in separating proven recommendations from unproven and perhaps unsafe claims.

*Your objectives in this chapter will be to:*

■ *Explain the uses of vitamins, minerals, and water in the body*

■ *Name food sources of principal vitamins and minerals*

■ *Evaluate your vitamin and mineral intake*

■ *List factors that affect the amount of a vitamin or mineral you need*

# VITAMINS: THE CONTROLLING SPARKS

Vitamins are substances that contain carbon but do not provide energy. They are needed in small amounts to control biological reactions within the body. The body is not able to produce these necessary substances or produces inadequate amounts, so we must find them in our diet.

Much of our current knowledge about vitamins and minerals has been learned from diseases caused by a *deficiency,* or a lack of a specific vitamin. Diseases that result from the dietary lack of one or more vitamins have been observed for centuries. Yet it was not until the early 1900s that scientists began to identify the link between these deficiency diseases and vital substances in food. Today there are 13 known vitamins that humans must consume in their diets to maintain health. No one natural food contains all the needed vitamins.

Initially scientists gave each new vitamin a letter name in order of its discovery (vitamin A was first, then vitamin B, and so on). Because vitamins are chemical compounds, often the chemical name, or scientific name, is used. For example, vitamin C is also known as ascorbic acid.

*Figure 4.1.*   In the past *beriberi,* a vitamin deficiency disease, occurred among people eating a diet consisting mainly of polished rice.

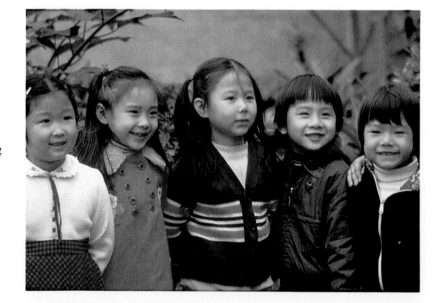

| Table 4.1    Vitamins are Classified by Solubility | |
| --- | --- |
| **Water-Soluble** | **Fat-Soluble** |
| Ascorbic Acid | Vitamin A |
| Thiamin | Vitamin D |
| Riboflavin | Vitamin E |
| Niacin | Vitamin K |
| Vitamin $B_6$ | |
| Folacin | |
| Vitamin $B_{12}$ | |
| Pantothenic Acid | |
| Biotin | |

Both natural and synthetic vitamins are present in today's food supply. *Natural* vitamins are those that occur naturally in food. *Synthetic* vitamins are produced in a scientific laboratory, then added to food products. Vitamin pills may contain either the natural or synthetic form of the vitamin. A vitamin's chemical structure, whether natural or synthetic, is the same. As a result, the body cannot tell the difference between them.

The 13 vitamins differ in their chemical structure and specific function. However, based on some common properties vitamins have been classified into two groups. Vitamins A, D, E, and K are labeled *fat-soluble,* because they mix with and are carried in dietary fats and oils. The remaining nine vitamins (vitamin C and the B complex vitamins) are *water-soluble*. Vitamins in each category have similar traits, making vitamin facts easier to remember and apply. See Table 4.1.

# FAT-SOLUBLE VITAMINS

Dietary fats and oils are sources of fat-soluble vitamins. The body absorbs these vitamins in a manner similar to fat absorption. Thus a person suffering from faulty fat absorption is likely to be lacking in fat-soluble vitamins. In the body, fat-soluble vitamins are stored in the liver and in fatty tissue. Therefore they need not be consumed daily. In fact, excess consumption of vitamins A and D may produce *toxic,* or poisonous, effects. Symptoms such as weight loss

**Table 4.2    Summary of Fat-Soluble Vitamins**

|  | **Vitamin A** | **Vitamin D** | **Vitamin E** | **Vitamin K** |
|---|---|---|---|---|
| Known Functions .... | Visual Purple<br>Normal Skin<br>and Mucous<br>Membranes<br>Bone Growth<br>Reproduction | Absorption of<br>Calcium<br>Normal Bone<br>Growth | Antioxidant | Normal Blood<br>Clotting |
| Vitamin Sources....... | Liver<br>Egg Yolk<br>Whole Milk<br>Dark Green and<br>Deep Orange<br>Vegetables | Sunshine<br>Fish Liver Oils<br>Fortified Milk<br>Egg Yolk | Wheat Germ<br>Vegetable Oils<br>Egg Yolk<br>Cereal Grains | Dark Green<br>Vegetables<br>Intestinal<br>Bacteria |
| Deficiency Symptoms ... | Night Blindness<br>Digestive<br>Disorders<br>Dry Skin<br>Respiratory<br>Infections | Rickets<br>Osteomalacia | None known to<br>occur in<br>adults<br>Red Blood Cell<br>Destruction in<br>Premature<br>Infants | Slower blood<br>clotting time<br>Hemorrhaging |
| Toxicity ......... | Headaches<br>Vomiting<br>Double Vision<br>Muscle and<br>Joint Pain | Vomiting<br>Weight Loss<br>Kidney<br>Damage | Headaches<br>Fatigue<br>Slower Blood<br>Clotting Time | Naturally<br>occurring<br>Vitamin K is<br>nontoxic<br>Excess Synthetic<br>Vitamin $K_3$<br>can produce<br>Red Blood<br>Cell and Liver<br>Damage |

and vomiting can be danger signals of excess vitamin intake. Fat-soluble vitamins are fairly stable when exposed to heat. Thus they are not readily destroyed during food processing, preservation, or preparation. See Table 4.2.

## Keep Your Eye on Vitamin A

"Eat your carrots and you'll see better in the dark" is a common saying. What do carrots have to do with eyesight? Carrots contain a pigment called *carotene*. This pigment is a *precursor* to vitamin A; in other words, vitamin A can be made from carotene. And vitamin A has a major function in the visual process.

The retina of the eye is sensitive to light. To see in dim light the retina produces a substance called *visual purple*. Vitamin A is a necessary part of visual purple. Bright light bleaches visual purple, so it must be reformed each time darkness is encountered. If the supply of vitamin A is inadequate, the formation of visual purple slows down. As a result, the eyes take longer to adjust to seeing in the dark. This disorder is known as *night blindness*. Long-term deficiency in vitamin A may produce an increasing loss of sight. See Illustration 4.1.

In addition, vitamin A plays a role in maintaining the health of cells that line the intestinal and respiratory tracts and that form the outer layer of skin. This normally smooth, moist tissue becomes dry and hard when vitamin A is lacking. Infection is more likely to occur when these cells are damaged. Although the details are not completely understood, vitamin A is also required for bone growth and normal reproduction.

The *active form* of the vitamin is only found in animal foods, such as milk, butter, egg yolk, and liver. Becauser the fat content is altered in low-fat and skim milk products, these must be *fortified* with vitamin A; in other words, vitamin A is added to these products after

*Illustration 4.1.* The Visual Process and Vitamin A.

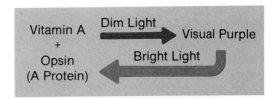

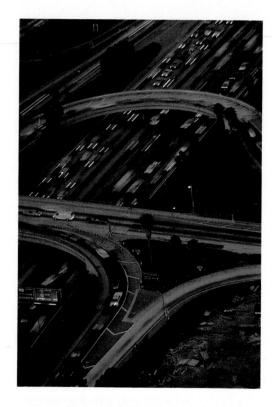

*Figure 4.2.* Night blindness can be caused by a shortage of vitamin A.

processing. Margarine is also fortified with vitamin A to provide a vitamin level similar to that of butter.

The vitamin's precursor, carotene, is found in plant products. It is converted to the active vitamin in the body. The yellow-orange color of fruits and vegetables is a clue to their carotene content. In addition, many dark green vegetables also contain carotene. Carrots, winter squash, cantaloupe, broccoli, and spinach are excellent sources of carotene.

Both active vitamin A and carotene may be present in the diet. The amount of the vitamin available from food is measured in *retinol equivalents*. Retinol is one of the active forms of vitamin A.

Do you know anyone whose skin has turned yellow-orange? It can happen! If it happens to you, it's time to reduce your carotene intake. Fortunately, excess carotene is not toxic. However, the effects of consuming too much active vitamin A can be serious. Headaches, vomiting, double vision, and muscle and joint pain are a few of the symptoms. Excessive intake of vitamin A is considered to be particularly dangerous to pregnant women, as birth defects may result.

If you are taking a vitamin supplement, choose one that provides carotene, the precursor form of vitamin A. Avoid high, daily doses or highly fortified foods unless prescribed by a doctor.

### Vitamin D: Let the Sun Shine

This unique vitamin may be obtained from food or from the action of the sun's rays on skin. The vitamin's chemical name is *calciferol*. Unlike other vitamins, it may be produced in the body by the action of sunlight on a cholesterol-like substance in the skin. The vitamin is then activated in the liver and kidney. However, many people do not receive adequate exposure to sunlight throughout the year. If dietary vitamin D is also lacking, a deficiency may occur. See Illustration 4.2.

Growing children are the most severely affected by the lack of vitamin D, as the vitamin is needed for normal formation of bones and teeth. A deficiency in children produces a disorder called *rickets,* in which the bones simply fail to calcify and harden. In adults the disorder is known as *osteomalacia*. See Illustration 4.3.

What foods are sources of vitamin D? Fish liver oils are the only excellent, naturally occurring food sources of vitamin D. Liver

*Figure 4.3.* Vitamin D is produced by the action of the sun's rays on the skin.

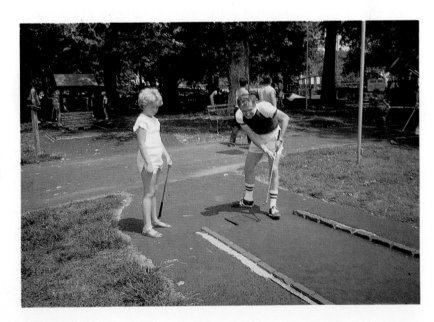

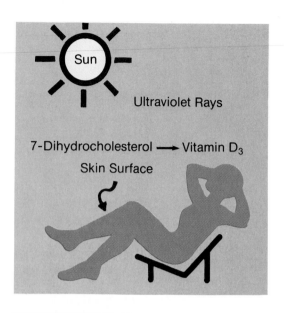

*Illustration 4.2.* Vitamin D: The Sunshine Vitamin.

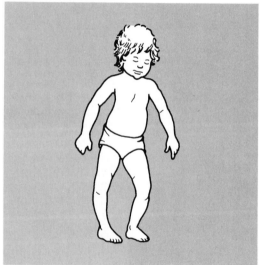

*Illustration 4.3.* Rickets: A Lack of Vitamin D.

and egg yolk are fair sources. Today, however, almost all milk has been fortified with vitamin D. Breast-fed infants and strict vegetarians should consume a vitamin D supplement.

Because the body stores vitamin D, excess intake may produce serious problems. Vomiting, weight loss, or kidney damage may result when the body receives more vitamin D than it needs.

## The Mysteries of Vitamin E

Vitamin E's chemical name, *tocopherol,* means "to bear offspring" in Greek. Although vitamin E is essential for fertility in rats, it does not play a major part in human reproduction. Popular press claims of vitamin E as a sex vitamin and an antiaging factor are, as yet, unproven by medical science. Its role in human nutrition remains controversial. Today, vitamin E is most widely recognized for its role as an *antioxidant.* This means the vitamin protects other substances, such as polyunsaturated fatty acids and vitamin A, from being destroyed by oxygen. The only known result of vitamin E deficiency is the destruction of red blood cells in premature infants.

Vitamin E is widely available in the American diet. Common food sources are vegetable oils, margarine, egg yolk, cereals, and legumes. The processing of white rice and refined flour decreases their vitamin E content.

Recent evidence suggests that excess vitamin E intake may interfere with vitamin K activity and prolong blood clotting time. Headaches and fatigue have also been associated with large doses of vitamin E. Hopefully, research into this vitamin will reveal its mysterious role in human nutrition.

## Vitamin K: Stop the Bleeding

Vitamin K is an essential factor in the clotting of blood. Without adequate vitamin K, a protein substance needed for blood clotting will not be formed. Therefore, the time taken for blood to

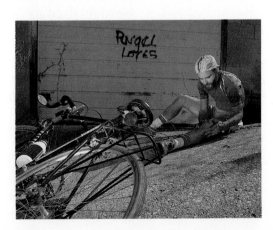

*Figure 4.4.*   Vitamin K is essential to the process of blood clotting.

form a clot will be longer, and *hemorrhaging,* or bleeding, will continue longer.

Bacteria in the intestine can synthesize about half the vitamin K humans need. The remainder must be obtained from the diet. Consumption of antibiotic drugs may decrease the amount of the vitamin produced by the intestinal bacteria. The best food sources of vitamin K are dark green vegetables, cabbage, and cauliflower. Meat and dairy products also are fair sources.

Three forms of vitamin K are known to exist. Vitamin $K_1$ occurs naturally in green plants. Vitamin $K_2$ is formed as a result of bacterial action in the intestinal tract. Scientists have also produced a synthetic form known as vitamin $K_3$. The synthetic form is twice as biologically active as the naturally occurring vitamin K. Excess vitamin $K_3$ can produce red blood cell and liver damage.

# WATER-SOLUBLE VITAMINS

The group of water-soluble vitamins is strikingly different from the fat-soluble vitamins. First, water-soluble vitamins are not stored to any extent in the body, so frequent and regular dietary intake is necessary. Second, when large amounts of a water-soluble vitamin are consumed, the excess is readily excreted. Toxic effects from overconsumption are less likely to occur.

Water-soluble vitamins are more easily destroyed by contact with heat, light, and basic substances, such as baking soda. See Table 4.3. They are also easily *leached,* or "soaked out of" foods prepared in water. The old adage, "Don't pour the vitamins down the drain," is based on the water solubility of these vitamins. Improper processing, preparation, and storage of foods may lower their water-soluble vitamin content.

## Ascorbic Acid (Vitamin C)

Will consuming extra vitamin C prevent or lessen the severity of the common cold? Scientific evidence is still sketchy, so the verdict is not in. In the meantime, what do nutrition scientists know about the body's need for ascorbic acid?

Ascorbic acid is needed for the development of connective tissue and to promote wound healing. Like vitamin E, ascorbic acid

## Table 4.3   Factors Affecting Stability of Water-Soluble Vitamins

| | Heat | Oxygen | Water Soaking | Alkali | Acid | Exposure to Light |
|---|---|---|---|---|---|---|
| Niacin | | | X | | | |
| Thiamin | X | X | X | X | | |
| Pyridoxine | X | | | X | | X |
| Folacin | X | | X | | X | |
| $B_{12}$ | | X | | X | X | X |
| Riboflavin | | | X | X | | X |
| Pantothenic Acid | X | | | X | X | |
| Biotin | | X | X | X | X | |
| Ascorbic Acid | X | X | X | X | | |

X = Unstable and vitamin activity loss in presence of factor.

serves as an antioxidant. It also enhances the body's absorption of the mineral *iron*. Cigarette smoking has been shown to increase the body's ascorbic acid requirement.

A deficiency of ascorbic acid results in *scurvy*. Scurvy plagued the New World explorers well into the 1800s. After months at sea the sailors would develop soft, bleeding gums and loose teeth. They also became weak and their skin bruised easily. In the mid 1700s, a British navy man named James Lind made a breakthrough. He found that scurvy could be cured by eating lemons and limes. Many years later the substance in limes that is responsible for curing scurvy was identified as ascorbic acid.

For many Americans, orange juice is the most frequently consumed source of ascorbic acid. Grapefruit, lemons, strawberries, broccoli, cabbage, and green pepper are also excellent sources. See Table 4.4.

## Thiamin (Vitamin $B_1$)

Scientists know today that eating foods high in carbohydrates increases the body's need for thiamin. Why? Thiamin, like all B vitamins, functions in the body as a coenzyme. (Recall that an enzyme speeds up a chemical reaction in the body.) Thiamin, as a coenzyme, is needed for the release of energy from carbohydrate. When energy

**Table 4.4    Ascorbic Acid Content of Selected Foods**

| Food | Serving Size | Ascorbic Acid Content (mg/serving) |
|---|---|---|
| Pepper, Sweet Green | 1 pepper | 94 |
| Orange Juice, frozen | 6 oz | 90 |
| Strawberries, fresh | 1 cup | 88 |
| Broccoli, fresh, cooked | 3 spears | 81 |
| Orange | 1 medium | 66 |
| Cantaloupe | ¼ melon | 45 |
| Grapefruit | ½ medium | 37 |
| Asparagus, cooked | ⅔ cup | 31 |
| Potato, white, baked | 1 medium | 31 |
| Tomato Juice, canned | 6 oz | 29 |
| Spinach, frozen, cooked | ½ cup | 27 |
| Winter Squash, mashed | 1 cup | 27 |
| Cabbage, cooked | ½ cup | 24 |
| Liver, Beef, cooked | 3 oz | 23 |
| Vegetable Juice Cocktail | 6 oz | 16 |
| Tomato, raw | ½ medium | 14 |
| Banana | 1 medium | 12 |
| Apricots, raw | 3 | 11 |

Source: United States Department of Agriculture, "Nutritive value of American Foods in Common Units" (Washington, D.C.: United States Government Printing Office, 1975), Handbook No. 456.

requirements are increased, such as during periods of growth or athletic activity, there is also a greater need for thiamin. In addition, thiamin is required for the breakdown of alcohol in the liver. Thiamin may also be involved in nerve function.

What are the effects of a diet lacking in thiamin? In the past, people surviving on a diet consisting primarily of polished (outer layer of kernel has been removed) white rice frequently developed muscle weakness and mental confusion. This disorder was known as *beriberi*. When the rice husks and bran were added back to their diets, the symptoms vanished. Eventually scientists isolated thiamin as the

## Table 4.5    Thiamin Content of Selected Foods

| Food | Serving Size | Thiamin Content (mg/serving) |
|---|---|---|
| Porkchop, lean, broiled......... | 3 oz | 0.92 |
| Ham, baked, lean ............... | 3 oz | 0.49 |
| Bran Flakes, 40% ............... | 1 cup | 0.41 |
| Peanuts, roasted, salted......... | ½ cup | 0.23 |
| Peas, frozen, cooked............ | ½ cup | 0.21 |
| Cashew Nuts, roasted........... | ⅓ cup | 0.20 |
| Asparagus, cooked.............. | ⅔ cup | 0.20 |
| Soybeans, cooked ............... | ½ cup | 0.19 |
| Oatmeal, cooked ................ | 1 cup | 0.19 |
| Orange Juice, frozen............ | 6 oz | 0.17 |
| Peas, Split, dried, cooked ........................ | ½ cup | 0.15 |
| Rice, white, cooked............. | ½ cup | 0.12 |
| Wheat Germ, toasted ........... | 1 tblsp | 0.11 |
| Yogurt, Nonfat Milk ............ | 1 cup | 0.11 |
| Milk, Low-fat, 2%.............. | 1 cup | 0.10 |
| Bread, Whole Wheat ........... | 1 slice | 0.06-0.09 |
| Broccoli, cooked ................ | ½ cup | 0.07 |
| Bread, White, enriched......... | 1 slice | 0.06 |

Source: United States Department of Agriculture, "Nutritive Value of American Foods in Common Units" (Washington, D.C.: United States Government Printing Office, 1975), Handbook No. 456.

substance missing from the diets of people with beriberi. Today alcoholism is the chief cause of thiamin deficiency.

Pork is the richest source of thiamin. As you might guess, thiamin is also found in whole grains and cereals. Today, food processors follow *enrichment* procedures, as they replace the thiamin lost in processing cereals, flour, and bread products. Read the product label, however, because by law only foods shipped between states must be enriched. Other good sources of thiamin include dried beans and peas, fresh green vegetables, and wheat germ. See Table 4.5.

Thiamin is easily dissolved in water, so only small amounts of water should be used in cooking vegetables. Steaming or microwaving

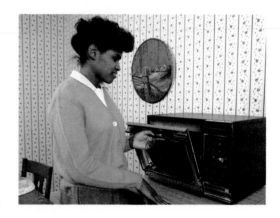

*Figure 4.5.* Vegetables cooked in a microwave retain their vitamin content.

vegetables preserves thiamin content, while cooking too long under pressure destroys the vitamin. The addition of baking soda will also make the vitamin inactive. The use of sulfur dioxide in drying fruits destroys their thiamin content. See Illustration 4.4.

### Riboflavin (Vitamin B$_2$)

As a coenzyme, riboflavin is needed for the release of energy from carbohydrates, fats, and proteins. Thus the amount of riboflavin needed in the diet is related to a person's energy needs and caloric intake.

The B vitamins appear in similar foods and often work with one another in the body. A separate deficiency disease has not been

*Illustration 4.4.* Using a Pressure Cooker or Baking Soda can result in Thiamin Loss.

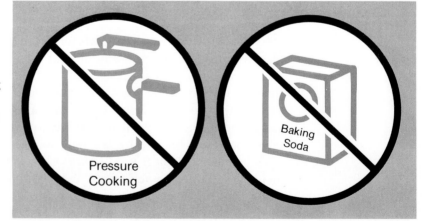

linked to riboflavin. However, a low intake does have visible effects, such as a purple tongue and a sore mouth with cracked skin at the corners. Growth retardation and very dry facial skin may also occur.

Many foods contain riboflavin, but in relatively small amounts. Milk and milk products are very good sources, as are meat and green leafy vegetables. Whole grain and enriched breads and cereals are fair sources of this vitamin. See Table 4.6. Although quite stable when exposed to heat, riboflavin may be lost in cooking water. In addition, the vitamin may be destroyed by sunlight. To protect the riboflavin content, milk should be packaged in a light-resistant container. See Illustration 4.5.

## Table 4.6    Riboflavin Content of Selected Foods

| Food | Serving Size | Riboflavin Content (mg/serving) |
|---|---|---|
| Milk, 2% | 8 oz | 0.52 |
| Yogurt, Low-Fat, plain | 8 oz | 0.49 |
| Bran Flakes, 40% | 1 cup | 0.49 |
| Milk, Whole | 1 cup | 0.41 |
| Yogurt, Low-Fat, flavored | 8 oz | 0.40 |
| Ice Cream, 10% fat | 1 cup | 0.28 |
| Porkchop, lean, broiled | 3 oz | 0.27 |
| Spinach, cooked | 1 cup | 0.25 |
| Asparagus, fresh, cooked | ⅔ cup | 0.22 |
| Cottage Cheese, uncreamed | ½ cup | 0.20 |
| Winter Squash, baked | ⅔ cup | 0.18 |
| Hamburger, 21% fat, cooked | 3 oz | 0.17 |
| Egg, Whole | 1 large | 0.15 |
| Broccoli, cooked | ⅔ cup | 0.15 |
| Cheddar Cheese | 1 oz | 0.13 |

Source: United States Department of Agriculture, "Nutritive Value of American Foods in Common Units" (Washington, D.C.: United States Government Printing Office, 1975), Handbook No. 456.

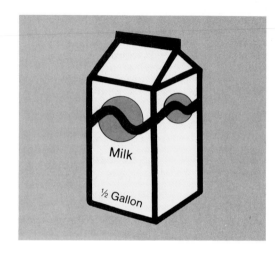

*Illustration 4.5.* Milk is Packaged in an Opaque Container to Preserve Riboflavin.

## Niacin (Vitamin B₃)

Niacin, or *nicotinic acid,* in its coenzyme form plays a role in the release of energy from carbohydrates, fats, and proteins. As a result, the amount needed by the body is in direct proportion to caloric intake.

In the early 1900s a disease of epidemic proportions hit the southeastern United States. Thousands of people sought treatment for symptoms of diarrhea, *dermatitis* (dry, scaly skin), and *dementia* (confusion and memory loss). Severe cases resulted in death. The disease was labeled *pellegra*. It was not caused by bacteria or a virus, however. The victims had one factor in common: a poor diet. Corn meal and salt pork comprised the major portion of the diet for many low-income people in the South. After much study, pellegra was linked to the lack of a vital dietary substance: *niacin*.

Foods rich in niacin include meat, poultry, fish, and legumes. See Table 4.7. Fruits, vegetables, grains, and dairy products contain much smaller amounts of niacin. In addition, the body is able to convert an amino acid, *tryptophan,* to niacin. A diet providing adequate protein will furnish an additional source of niacin. Thus the niacin available in the diet is measured in *niacin equivalents.*

## Table 4.7    Niacin Content of Selected Foods

| Food | Serving Size | Niacin Content (mg/serving) |
|------|------|------|
| Round Steak | 3 oz | 5.1 |
| Chicken | 2 pieces | 5.8 |
| Peanut Butter | 1 tblsp | 2.4 |
| Beans, Pinto | ½ cup | 2.1 |
| Bran Muffin | 1 muffin | 1.7 |
| Cornmeal | ½ cup | 1.2 |
| Banana | 1 medium | 0.8 |
| Bread, Whole Wheat | 1 slice | 0.8 |
| Bread, White, enriched | 1 slice | 0.6 |
| Orange | 1 medium | 0.5 |
| Milk, Whole | 1 cup | 0.2 |

Source: United States Department of Agriculture, "Nutritive Value of American Foods in Common Units" (Washington, D.C.: United States Government Printing Office, 1975), Handbook No. 456.

## Vitamin B$_6$

Here's an exception to the rule. Recent medical findings indicate that large doses of this water-soluble vitamin may be toxic. Symptoms of toxicity include difficulty walking, numbness of feet and hands, and facial paralysis. What makes this vitamin unique? Vitamin B$_6$ is actually a complex of three chemically related compounds. The vitamin's major role is as a coenzyme. But instead of energy release, it is required for the breakdown and building of amino acids.

Because the body needs vitamin B$_6$ for efficient use of protein, the amount required parallels protein intake. A lack of the vitamin results in a form of *anemia* in which the red blood cells are pale and smaller than normal. Symptoms may include weakness, irritability, and sleeplessness. There appears to be an increased need for the vitamin during pregnancy and with the use of birth control pills. In addition, heavy alcohol intake hinders the body's ability to use vitamin B$_6$.

**Table 4.8  Vitamin B$_6$ Content of Selected Foods**

| Food | Serving Size | Vitamin B$_6$ Content (mg/serving) |
|---|---|---|
| Liver, Beef, fried.............. | 3 oz | 0.569 |
| Banana......................... | 1 medium | 0.480 |
| Avocado ....................... | ½ medium | 0.420 |
| Hamburger, cooked ........... | 3 oz | 0.391 |
| Chicken, fried ................ | 3 oz | 0.340 |
| Corn, cooked .................. | ½ cup | 0.246 |
| Potato, White, baked in skin.......................... | 1 medium | 0.200 |
| Spinach, cooked............... | ½ cup | 0.161 |
| Haddock, fried................. | 3½ oz | 0.140 |
| Peas, Green, cooked.......... | ½ cup | 0.110 |
| Broccoli, cooked .............. | ½ cup | 0.107 |
| Milk, Whole ................... | 1 cup | 0.098 |
| Bread, Whole Wheat ......... | 1 slice | 0.041 |
| Rice, White, enriched, cooked ...................... | ½ cup | 0.030 |

Source: Adapted from: J. A. Pennington, "Dietary Nutrient Guide," copyright 1976 by AVI Publishing Company, Westport, Connecticut.

Vitamin B$_6$ is widely available in food, but often in small quantities. The best sources include yeast, organ and muscle meats, bananas, and whole grain products. The vitamin is heat resistant, but losses do occur when it is exposed to sunlight and baking soda. See Table 4.8.

## Folacin

The term folacin refers to several active forms of the vitamin, including folic acid. Folacin is required for normal cell division and building protein tissue in the body. Thus the need for the vitamin increases during pregnancy, periods of growth, and illness. See Illustration 4.6.

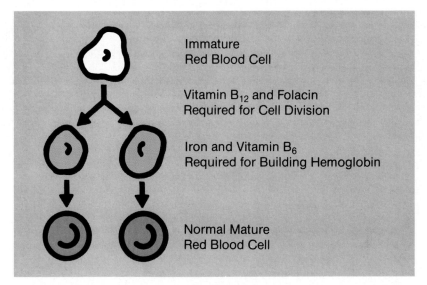

***Illustration 4.6.*** Vitamins and Minerals Involved in Red Blood Cell Production.

Immature
Red Blood Cell

Vitamin $B_{12}$ and Folacin
Required for Cell Division

Iron and Vitamin $B_6$
Required for Building Hemoglobin

Normal Mature
Red Blood Cell

 

A deficiency of folacin results in another form of anemia. In this case both red and white blood cells are much larger than normal. Other effects include a slowing of growth and changes in the tissues that line the intestine. Alcohol and some prescription drugs may reduce the absorption of folacin and contribute to a deficiency.

Food sources of folacin include green leafy vegetables, organ meats, nuts, legumes, and yeast. The vitamin is quickly destroyed by heat, so cooking loss may be considerable. See Table 4.9.

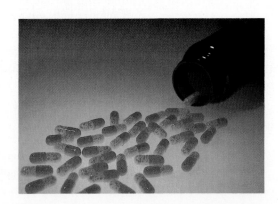

***Figure 4.6.*** Certain prescription drugs hinder nutrient absorption.

### Table 4.9    Folacin Content of Selected Foods

| Food | Serving Size | Folacin Content ($\mu$g/serving) |
|---|---|---|
| Yeast, Brewers .............. | 1 Tblsp | 313 |
| Liver, Beef, cooked ........ | 3 oz | 123 |
| Spinach, raw ............... | 1 cup | 106 |
| Orange Juice ............... | 6 oz | 102 |
| Orange, raw ................ | 1 medium | 65 |
| Broccoli, cooked .......... | ½ cup | 44 |
| Beans, Red, cooked ........ | ½ cup | 34 |
| Banana ..................... | 1 medium | 33 |
| Egg, whole, raw ........... | 1 medium | 29 |
| Yogurt ...................... | 1 cup | 27 |
| Wheat Germ................. | 1 Tblsp | 20 |
| Lettuce, head or leaf ....... | 1 cup | 20 |
| Bread, Whole Wheat....... | 1 slice | 16 |
| Shredded Wheat ........... | 1 oz | 14 |
| Peanut Butter............... | 1 Tblsp | 13 |

Source: Adapted from B. P. Perloff and R. R. Butrum, "Folacin in Selected Foods," *Journal of the American Dietetic Association* 70 (1977): 161.

## Vitamin $B_{12}$

Vitamin $B_{12}$, as a coenzyme, functions along with folacin in promoting normal cell division. A lack of vitamin $B_{12}$ also produces an anemia with enlarged blood cells. A vitamin $B_{12}$ deficiency affects the functioning of the nervous system.

Adequate intake is not the only problem resulting in $B_{12}$ deficiency. In order to be absorbed, vitamin $B_{12}$ must be bound to a protein produced in the stomach known as *intrinsic factor*. Vitamin $B_{12}$ and intrinsic factor work together like a lock and key. If you do not have the right key, the door cannot be opened. Similarly, without the intrinsic factor vitamin $B_{12}$ cannot cross the lining of the small intestine and enter the bloodstream. If this intrinsic factor is absent, *pernicious anemia* results. This anemia is treated by giving injections or massive oral doses of vitamin $B_{12}$.

### Table 4.10    Vitamin B$_{12}$ Content of Selected Foods

| Food | Serving Size | B$_{12}$ Content ($\mu$g/serving) |
|---|---|---|
| Liver, Beef, cooked........ | 3 oz | 68 |
| Oysters, canned ........... | 3½ oz | 18 |
| Lamb Leg, roasted........ | 3 oz | 2.63 |
| Tuna, canned............... | 2 oz | 1.32 |
| Yogurt, Low-Fat........... | 8 oz | 1.06 |
| Skim Milk.................. | 8 oz | 0.946 |
| Milk, Whole ............... | 8 oz | 0.871 |
| Egg, Whole ................ | 1 large | 0.773 |
| Cottage Cheese............ | ½ cup | 0.704 |
| Halibut, broiled ........... | 3 oz | 0.85 |
| Pork, roasted............... | 3 oz | 0.42 |
| Chicken, roasted .......... | 3 oz | 0.36 |

Source: From T. A. Pennington, "Dietary Nutrient Guide," copyright 1976, AVI Publishing Company, Westport, Connecticut.

Strict vegetarians need to pay special attention to vitamin B$_{12}$. This vitamin is found only in foods of animal origin. Organ and muscle meats, seafood, eggs, and milk are the major food sources. See Table 4.10.

### Less Familiar B Vitamins

Pantothenic acid and biotin are the remaining B vitamins. Both vitamins function as coenzymes.

***Pantothenic Acid.*** This vitamin is a component of a critical coenzyme needed for production of energy. A lack of this vitamin is rare, but a deficiency can produce fatigue and numbness and tingling in the feet and hands. Food sources of the vitamin include yeast, organ meats, bran, peanuts, and mushrooms.

***Biotin.*** Biotin is involved in building fatty acids. Biotin deficiency is rare, but may be caused by consuming large amounts of raw eggs. A protein in the raw egg binds with biotin, preventing absorption. Symptoms of deficiency are dry, scaly skin, muscle pain, and nausea. Bacteria in the body are able to produce some biotin. Milk and milk products are the best dietary sources.

# MINERALS: THE CRITICAL BALANCE

Just as minerals provide structure and add strength to skyscrapers and airplanes, some are also vital components of the human body. Minerals, such as iron, copper, and zinc, are inorganic, or non-carbon-containing elements. These substances are mined from the earth's crust for industrial use. However, the minerals needed by the body are present in the food and water we consume. In fact, about 4% of the body's weight is minerals.

Of the 60 known minerals, only about one third are known to be essential to human health. Minerals have different functions in the body. However, many work together and with other nutrients to accomplish their tasks. A safe and effective, functioning mineral balance in the body is vital. For this reason, eating too much of a mineral is as much of a problem as eating too little.

Minerals are needed by the body in relatively small amounts. Minerals present in the body in fairly large amounts are classified as *major minerals*. Those found in much smaller amounts are known as *trace minerals*. Both groups are equally important to maintaining internal balance. See Table 4.11.

# MAJOR MINERALS

## Calcium

As a child you were told to drink your milk for strong bones and teeth. Actually, the minerals present in milk, calcium and phosphorus, are the necessary elements for bone and tooth development. *Calcium* accounts for about 2 to 3 pounds of your body weight. Almost 99% of the body's calcium is found in bone. However, the need for dietary calcium is not limited to periods of growth. The remaining calcium, found in body fluids, is crucial for normal muscle

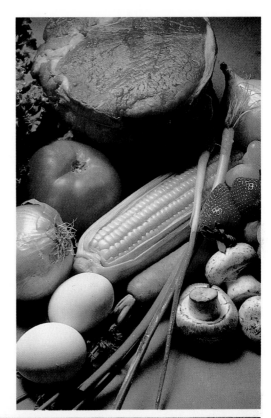

*Figure 4.7*.   Minerals such as iron and zinc can be mined from the earth. Found also in food and water, they are essential to a healthy body.

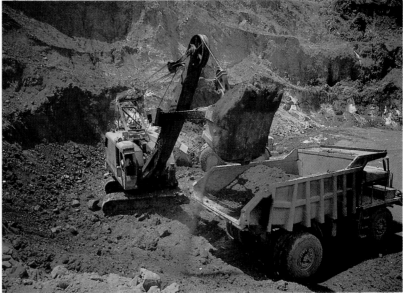

| Table 4.11    Classification of Minerals | |
|---|---|
| **Major Minerals** | **Trace Minerals** |
| Calcium | Iron |
| Phosphorus | Zinc |
| Chlorine | Fluorine |
| Potassium | Copper |
| Sulfur | Iodine |
| Sodium | Manganese |
| Magnesium | Selenium |
| | Molybdenum |
| | Chromium |
| | Silicon[a] |
| | Cobalt[a] |
| | Nickel[a] |
| | Vanadium[a] |
| | Tin[a] |
| | Arsenic[a] |
| | Cadmium[a] |

[a]Scientific evidence indicates that these minerals may be essential.

contractions, blood clotting, nerve impulses, and maintenance of cell collagen.

Bone, once formed, is not inert. The calcium stored in bone is slowly but constantly drawn out and redeposited as the level of blood calcium falls and rises. This process is controlled by *hormones,* substances that stimulate internal activities in response to the body's needs. See Illustration 4.7.

The need for calcium is proportionately greater for children undergoing rapid growth than for adults. However, loss of calcium from the bone is a problem for the elderly. Thus adequate calcium intake is important throughout life. Although an individual may consume enough calcium, other factors, such as stress and exercise, can alter the amount of calcium used by the body.

A calcium deficiency becomes evident only after severe loss of calcium from the bone. *Osteoporosis,* a decrease in the amount of bone in the body, plagues millions of older adults, particularly

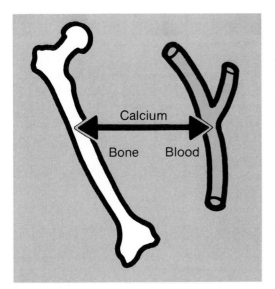

***Illustration 4.7.*** Calcium Regulation. Many factors affect the slow, constant exchange of calcium between bones and blood.

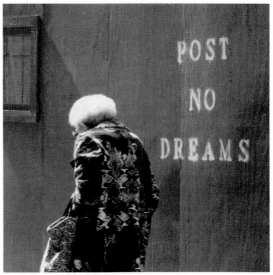

***Figure 4.8.*** *Osteoporosis,* a decrease in the amount of bone mass in the body, is a problem for many older adults:

women. Several factors are believed to contribute to the development of the disorder. These include hormone imbalance, poor calcium absorption, decreased physical activity, and high protein and phosphorus intakes. *Demineralization,* or loss of calcium and phosphorus from the bones, is known as *osteomalacia.* This disease is thought to be produced by a lack of vitamin D. *Rickets* is a comparable disorder in children. However, inadequate intake or an imbalance in calcium and phosphorus may also contribute to these diseases.

Milk and milk products are the primary dietary sources of calcium. See Table 4.12. In addition, broccoli, dark green leafy vegetbles, dried peas and beans, shellfish, and canned fish with edible bones are good sources. Not all food sources of calcium are equally available for absorption. For example, cocoa, rhubarb, and some green leafy vegetables, such as spinach, contain *oxalic acid.* This substance binds with calcium in the intestine, limiting calcium absorption. Another substance, *phytic acid,* found in legumes and grain also hinders calcium absorption.

## Table 4.12  Calcium Content of Selected Foods

| Food | Serving Size | Calcium Content (mg/serving) |
|---|---|---|
| Sardines | 3 oz | 372 |
| Milk, 2% | 1 cup | 352 |
| Salmon, Red, canned | 3½ oz | 285 |
| Yogurt | 1 cup | 272 |
| Turnip Greens, cooked | 1 cup | 267 |
| Cheddar Cheese | 1 oz | 204 |
| Tofu | 2″ square | 154 |
| Collard Greens | ½ cup | 145 |
| Pancakes | 2 | 100 |
| Cottage Cheese | ½ cup | 100 |
| Spinach, cooked | ½ cup | 100 |
| Ice Cream, 10% fat | ½ cup | 88 |
| Soybeans, cooked | ½ cup | 66 |
| Molasses, medium | 1 tblsp | 58 |
| Bran Muffin | 1 muffin | 57 |
| Orange, raw | 1 | 54 |
| Bread, White | 1 slice | 21 |

Source: United States Department of Agriculture, "Nutritive Value of American Foods in Common Units" (Washington, D.C.: United States Government Printing Office, 1975), Handbook No. 456.

## Phosphorus

Less popularized but just as important in bone formation is phosphorus. Phosphorus and calcium combine for added skeletal strength. About 85% of the body's phosphorus is present in bone and teeth. However, lesser quantities are present in every cell in the body. Phosphorus is required for cells to transfer and store energy. It also acts as a buffer in the blood, thus regulating the body's acid-base balance.

Phosphorus is abundant in our food supply. Foods high in protein, such as meat, milk, and eggs, contain significant amounts of phosphorus. Thus a diet adequate in protein supplies sufficient

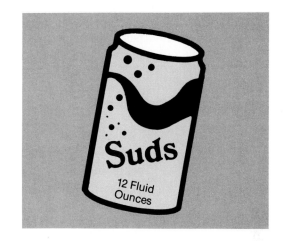

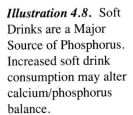

***Illustration 4.8.*** Soft Drinks are a Major Source of Phosphorus. Increased soft drink consumption may alter calcium/phosphorus balance.

phosphorus. The dietary requirement for phosphorus parallels that of calcium. In fact, consuming an equal ratio is desirable, because a very high phosphorus intake will tip the normal calcium-phosphorus balance. For example, soft drinks contain significant amounts of phosphorus, unaccompanied by calcium. Frequent consumption of soft drinks may disturb this balance. See Illustration 4.8. Milk products contain approximately equal amounts of calcium and phosphorus, so drinking more milk will not offset the imbalance. Because it is difficult to find foods that increase only calcium intake, too many soft drinks should be avoided.

## Magnesium

Bone is also the storage site of about 70% of the body's magnesium. The remainder is present in soft tissue and blood. In cells, magnesium assists phosphorus in the storage of readily available chemical energy. The presence of magnesium also triggers muscle to relax after calcium has stimulated contraction. Thus these minerals work together for proper functioning of the heart, nervous system, and skeletal muscles.

Magnesium deficiency is rare, but may occur as a result of alcoholism or prolonged vomiting and diarrhea. Severe muscle contraction and convulsions are symptoms of deficiency.

Food sources high in magnesium include nuts, dried beans and peas, whole grains, cereals, seafood, and chocolate. Only about half of the magnesium we consume is absorbed.

## Sodium

Table salt, or *sodium chloride,* is the most visible source of sodium in the diet. See Illustration 4.9. Sodium comprises 40% of this compound by weight. Thus 1 teaspoon of salt contains 2132 milligrams of sodium. Sodium plays a role in nerve impulse, acid-base balance, and the metabolism of carbohydrates and proteins. See Illustration 4.10.

Normally, 50% of the sodium in the body is present in the fluid outside the cells. In solution, sodium (as well as potassium and chloride) have the ability to take on electrical charges. Electrically charged particles are calls *ions*. As a positive ion, sodium exerts a major force in regulating body water balance. Because sodium intake varies daily, the kidneys must maintain a constant internal level by retaining or excreting sodium.

In some people this control mechanism fails to work properly. If excess sodium is retained in the body, extra water is also retained. As a result, the blood volume increases, along with blood pressure. Thus a person at risk for *hypertension,* or high blood pressure, is advised to limit his or her sodium intake.

***Illustration 4.9.*** Sodium Content of Table Salt.

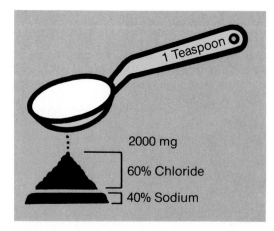

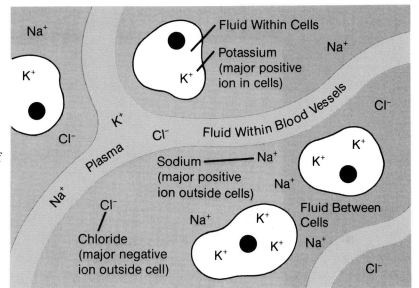

***Illustration 4.10.*** Sodium, Potassium, and Chlorine: Regulators of Body Water Balance.

In addition to table salt, sodium is widely available in food, beverages, and health products. Drinking water varies in natural sodium, with softened water containing a higher sodium content. See Table 4.13. Many foods are preserved or flavored with salt or salt brine, such as pickles, sauerkraut, olives, and cured and smoked meats. Other foods high in sodium include canned soups and vegetables and snack items such as chips, crackers, and pretzels. Sources of sodium often overlooked by the consumer include monosodium glutamate (MSG), soy sauce, baking soda, sodium saccharin, sodium benzoate, and sodium nitrate. You will even find sodium in toothpaste and antacids. Thus reading the ingredient label is a habit worth developing.

## Potassium

As a positive ion, potassium works closely with sodium to control the body's fluid balance. Unlike sodium, potassium is found almost entirely inside body cells. Nerve and muscle cells are particularly rich in potassium. In addition to maintaining fluid

## Table 4.13   Sodium Content of Selected Foods

| Food | Serving Size | Sodium Content (mg/serving) |
|---|---|---|
| Garlic Salt..................... | 1 tsp | 1850 |
| Meat Tenderizer.............. | 1 tsp | 1750 |
| Chicken Noodle Soup, canned..................... | 1 cup | 1152 |
| Ham.......................... | 3 oz | 1114 |
| Soy Sauce.................... | 1 tblsp | 1029 |
| Baked Beans, canned ....... | 1 cup | 928 |
| Pickles, Dill ................. | 1 pickle | 928 |
| Tomato Juice, canned ....... | 1 cup | 878 |
| Baking Soda ................. | 1 tsp | 821 |
| Frankfurter................... | 1 frankfurter | 639 |
| Cheese, American, processed.................. | 1 oz | 406 |
| Tuna, canned in oil.......... | 3 oz | 303 |
| Bacon, cooked .............. | 2 slices | 274 |
| Salad Dressing, French ..... | 1 tblsp | 214 |
| Catsup ...................... | 1 tblsp | 156 |
| Milk, Low-Fat............... | 1 cup | 122 |

Source: United States Department of Agriculture (Washington, D.C.: United States Government Printing Office), Home and Garden Bulletin No. 233.

balance, potassium enhances protein synthesis, muscle contraction, and nerve impulses. The mineral also plays a role in carbohydrate metabolism.

As with sodium, the kidneys control the amount of potassium retained in the body. There is a narrow margin of safety between too little and too much. Excess potassium loss may occur through heavy perspiration, persistent diarrhea, and use of diuretics. A lack of potassium produces nausea, muscle weakness, and rapid heart beat. An excess intake in tablet form is unwise, because this increases the work of the kidney to excrete the mineral to maintain a safe blood level. If the kidney fails to excrete the excess, mental confusion, numbness, breathing problems, and irregular heart beat may result.

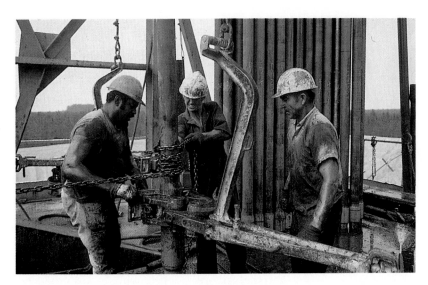

*Figure 4.9.* Heavy perspiration can cause an excessive loss of sodium and potassium.

Potassium is widely distributed in foods. Citrus fruits, bananas, potatoes, tomatoes, and dried fruits are particularly good sources. Meat and milk products also contain fair amounts of potassium.

## Chlorine

The majority of chlorine is present in the body as the negative ion *chloride*. Chloride is primarily found in fluids outside the cell. Working with sodium and potassium, chloride assists in maintaining normal fluid balance. As a component of *hydrochloric acid,* chlorine maintains normal stomach acidity. This acid medium aids in the digestion of proteins and vitamin $B_{12}$. A loss of chloride, such as through vomiting, can alter the body's acid-base balance. Sodium chloride (table salt) is the most common dietary source of chlorine.

## Sulfur

Sulfur, as a component of several amino acids, is present in all body cells. The vitamins thiamin and biotin contain sulfur. Sulfur is most abundant in skin and hair tissue and as a component of insulin. Sulfur is obtained in the diet primarily from foods high in protein.

## TRACE MINERALS

Trace minerals are the focus of much of the current nutritional research. These minerals are present in minute quantities in the body. Scientists have only recently developed the equipment necessary to study their presence and role in human nutrition. Equally important is determination of the best nutritional requirements of each. Some trace minerals are extremely toxic in larger quantities. In addition, trace minerals appear to function best in proportion to one another. Thus supplementing your diet with one trace mineral could proportionately decrease the presence of another.

Generally, trace minerals function as parts of body compounds, enzymes, vitamins, and hormones. Their presence in the diet depends on the mineral content of the soil in which the food was grown. Where do the foods you eat come from? Today the supermarket shelves are stocked with foods produced throughout the hemisphere. Mineral deficiencies are unlikely with such a diverse food supply. However, food processing frequently removes valuable trace elements. Thus a diet that relies heavily on processed foods may be inadequate in trace minerals.

*Figure 4.10.* The soil in which food is grown determines the amount of trace minerals in the food eaten.

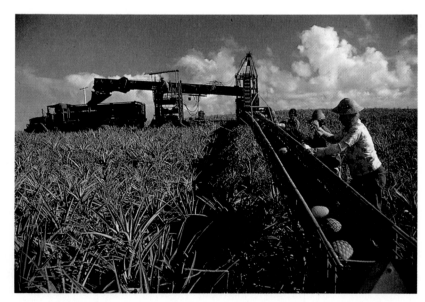

## Iron

The major role iron plays in the body is as a component of *hemoglobin,* an iron-containing protein. Hemoglobin, present in red blood cells, is responsible for the transport of oxygen to the cells. Iron serves a similar purpose in *myoglobin,* a muscle protein. In addition, iron is a part of several enzymes and is involved in protein synthesis.

The life of a red blood cell is about 120 days, so new hemoglobin is continually being formed. However, the body efficiently recycles iron and very little is excreted. In fact, the body does not have a way of excreting excess iron. Instead, the intestine controls the amount absorbed. When iron stores are low, absorption of dietary iron increases. There are two forms of dietary iron. Iron exists as an *organic* compound in red blood cells and muscle tissue. Eating meat provides us with organic iron. Organic iron is most readily absorbed. Iron, in its mineral or *inorganic* form, is found in both animal and plant foods. Absorption of inorganic iron is enhanced by an acid medium in the intestine. See Illustration 4.11. For example, drinking orange juice with a peanut butter sandwich increases iron absorption. A diet high in fiber and phytic acid will hinder absorption.

As a component of blood, iron is lost whenever there is blood loss. Thus women, needing to replace menstrual loss, have a greater need for iron. The need for iron is also greater when the number of red blood cells is increasing, such as during pregnancy, infancy, and the teenage growth spurt.

Low intake, poor absorption, and excess blood loss can decrease the body's iron reserves. When iron stores are low, the synthesis of hemoglobin is reduced. *Iron deficiency anemia,* with

***Illustration 4.11.*** Iron Absorption is Increased in the Presence of an Acid.

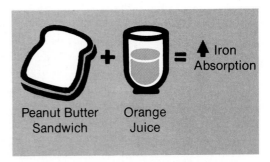

## Table 4.14    Iron Content of Selected Foods

| Foods | Serving Size | Iron Content (mg/serving) |
|---|---|---|
| Bran Flakes | 1 cup | 12.0 |
| Liver, Beef | 3 oz | 7.5 |
| Molasses, Blackstrap | 1 tblsp | 3.2 |
| Prune Juice | ½ cup | 5.2 |
| Hamburger | 3 oz | 2.6 |
| Red Kidney Beans, cooked | ½ cup | 2.2 |
| Spinach, cooked | ½ cup | 2.1 |
| Shredded Wheat | 1 cup | 1.8 |
| Raisins | 1½ oz | 1.5 |
| Bread, Whole Wheat | 1 slice | 0.8 |
| Banana | 1 medium | 0.8 |
| Bread, White, enriched | 1 slice | 0.6 |
| Orange | 1 medium | 0.6 |
| Broccoli, cooked | ½ cup | 0.6 |

Source: United States Department of Agriculture, "Nutritive Value of American Foods in Common Units" (Washington, D.C.: United States Government Printing Office, 1975), Handbook No. 456.

small, pale red blood cells, may result. Excess intake of iron may produce toxic effects, including liver and kidney damage.

Foods high in iron include liver, red meats, dried beans, whole grain and enriched breads and cereals, and dried fruits. Dark green vegetables are also good sources, although less is absorbed. The iron in egg yolk is also poorly absorbed. See Table 4.14.

## Iodine

Iodine is a component of two hormones produced by the thyroid gland. These hormones regulate growth and the basal metabolic rate. A lack of iodine produces a *goiter,* or visibly enlarged thyroid gland. See Illustration 4.12. The goiter occurs because the

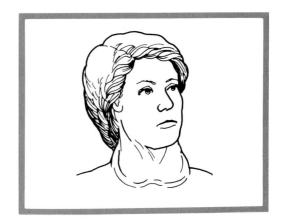

*Illustration 4.12*. A Goiter Develops from Lack of Iodine.

thyroid must increase its activity and size to offset the decline in iodine. Iodine deficiency has occurred in areas where soil was lacking iodine and the food supply was primarily regional.

Good sources of iodine include fish, seafood, and seaweed. However, salt has been iodized to provide an inexpensive and uniform source of iodine for all consumers. Today, scientists worry about the possibility of too much iodine in our food supply. One unexpected source has been milk, since bulk tanks are cleaned with an iodine solution.

## Copper

Copper is present throughout the body, but it is particularly concentrated in the liver, kidneys, heart, and brain. Copper is a component of several enzymes and is needed for the effective use of iron. Loss of taste, kinky hair, and nerve and skeletal breakdown may result from a lack of copper. Most often copper imbalance is caused by a genetic defect.

Foods high in copper include nuts, raisins, liver, legumes, and shellfish. Its content in drinking water will vary with water hardness.

## Fluorine

Does your toothpaste contain fluoride? No doubt you have heard the commercials promising fewer cavities with fluoridated

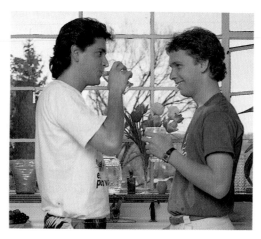

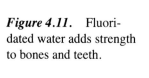
*Figure 4.11.* Fluoridated water adds strength to bones and teeth.

toothpaste. Although scientists have not confirmed a specific metabolic role for fluorine, it appears that its ion *fluoride* adds strength to bones and teeth. The reduction of *caries,* or tooth decay, has been achieved by drinking fluoridated water, using a fluoride mouth rinse, and applying fluoride to the tooth surface.

Food sources of fluoride are variable. The fluoride content of drinking water also varies. Thus many communities with low fluoride levels have chosen to fluoridate their water supply. Some water supplies have very high natural fluoride content. High levels of fluoride cause *mottling,* or discoloration, of the teeth, but this is not harmful.

## Zinc

In the body zinc functions as a component of the hormone, insulin. Numerous enzymes also contain zinc. In addition, it is needed for the synthesis of proteins and collagen. The role of zinc in human nutrition continues to be studied. Scientists have linked a lack of zinc to delays in growth and sexual development. Also, taste and wound healing are believed to be impaired when the zinc supply is inadequate.

Food sources of zinc include nuts, legumes, shellfish, and whole grains.

## Table 4.15    Summary of Trace Mineral Function and Sources

| Mineral | Function | Food Sources |
|---|---|---|
| Iron | An essential part of hemoglobin, to carry oxygen to body via the red blood cells; lack of iron can cause anemia | Liver, red meats, dried beans and peas, enriched or whole grain breads and cereals, prunes, raisins |
| Iodine | Forms part of hormones of thyroid gland, which helps regulate body metabolism; lack can cause goiter | Iodized salt, seafood, plants grown near sea |
| Zinc | Needed for tissue repair and normal growth of skeleton; part of several hormones, including insulin; involved in cell metabolism | Red meat, milk, liver, seafood, eggs, whole grain or fortified cereal |
| Fluoride | Helps prevent dental caries; helps stabilize bones and teeth; deficiency can cause tooth decay, osteoporosis | Fluoridated drinking water best source |
| Copper | Vital to enzyme system and in manufacturing red blood cells; need for utilization of iron; anemia possible, but deficiencies are rare | Oysters, nuts, liver, kidney, whole grain breads and cereals, mushrooms |
| Manganese | Vital to various enzyme systems involved in protein and energy metabolism; essential for normal bone structure and functioning of central nervous system | Nuts, whole grain breads and cereals, tea, vegetables, fruits |

*(Continued)*

Source: C. Lecos, "Tracking Trace Minerals," *FDA Consumer* (Washington, D.C.: United States Government Printing Office, 1983), HHS Publication No. (FDA) 83-2176.

**Table 4.15 (cont'd)**

| Mineral | Function | Food Sources |
|---|---|---|
| Chromium | Essential for normal glucose metabolism; helps regulate insulin levels | Brewer's yeast, cheese, whole grains, meat |
| Selenium | Essential role in enzyme systems of animals and proper functioning of blood | Varied diet provides adequate amounts—fish, meat, breads, cereals |
| Molybdenum | Essential to function of enzymes involved in production of uric acid and in oxidation of sulfites and aldehydes | Meats, grains, legumes |

### The Remaining Trace Minerals

Of the remaining trace elements, specific roles have been identified for chromium, manganese, selenium, and molybdenum. *Chromium* appears to be necessary for the body to store and use glucose. Scientists believe it may act as a cofactor of insulin. *Manganese* is an essential part of several enzymes related to energy and protein metabolism. As a part of an enzyme, *selenium* protects cells from being destroyed by oxygen. *Molybdenum* is also known to be needed for enzyme function. See Table 4.15.

The roles, if any, of silicon, cobalt, nickel, vanadium, tin, arsenic, and cadmium are still under study.

## PUTTING THE NUTRIENT PUZZLE TOGETHER

As you can see, there are many pieces to the nutrition puzzle. Until now the focus has been on individual nutrients, their roles and food sources. If this seems a bit overwhelming to you, you're not alone! What should be most evident is that a nutritionally adequate diet must include a variety of foods. Eating is a part of your daily routine. How can you ensure nutrient adequacy and balance in your diet? The next chapter will offer practical advice for planning and evaluating your food intake.

## CHECK YOUR PROGRESS

1. What is the general function of a vitamin in the body?
2. How many vitamins are currently known to be essential to humans?
3. Can your body tell the difference between natural and synthetic vitamins?
4. List the fat-soluble and water-soluble vitamins. Explain why water-soluble vitamins need to be consumed daily. Why is it not a good idea to consume large quantities of fat-soluble vitamins?
5. What is a precursor?
6. What is the precursor of vitamin A? Name some of its food sources. What foods are sources of active vitamin A?
7. What is the chemical name of vitamin D? Describe two ways you can obtain this vitamin.
8. Name the disorder that occurs in children who are lacking in vitamin D. Name the similar disorder that occurs in adults.
9. Identify the main function of vitamin E. Name several food sources of vitamin E.
10. Why does the body need vitamin K? Name a food source of vitamin K. How else does the body obtain this vitamin?
11. Explain how the water-soluble vitamin content of a food might be destroyed.
12. What is another name for vitamin C? Cite several food sources of this vitamin.
13. Name the deficiency disease that occurs when vitamin C intake is inadequate. What are its symptoms?
14. Explain why your need for thiamin rises as your energy requirements increase.
15. What disorder occurs when the diet is lacking in thiamin? Give an example of a thiamin-rich food.
16. Name the deficiency disease with symptoms of diarrhea, dermatitis, and dementia. Identify which vitamin is lacking.

17. Identify the amino acid that can be converted to niacin.
18. Name the vitamin required for the breaking down and building up of protein. What foods are sources of this vitamin?
19. A form of anemia with enlarged red and white blood cells results from a lack of which vitamin? Name common food sources of the vitamin.
20. Name the vitamin that is found only in foods of animal origin. What substance, produced in the stomach, is required for the absorption of this vitamin? Identify the disease that results if this substance is lacking.
21. Explain why consuming too much of any one mineral is as much of a problem as consuming too little.
22. List the major minerals. List the trace minerals.
23. Describe the roles of calcium in the body. Identify the main food source of this mineral. What disorder, common in older women, is related to calcium intake?
24. In addition to calcium, what other mineral is required for bone strength? Why are researchers concerned about this mineral in people who frequently consume soft drinks?
25. How does the body use magnesium? Name several food sources.
26. Define ion.
27. What is the main source of sodium in the diet? Explain the major role of sodium in the body. What happens when excess sodium is retained in the body?
28. Name the other positively charged mineral that works with sodium to regulate fluid balance. What events might cause excess loss of this mineral from the body?
29. Identify the principal negatively charged mineral involved in fluid balance. What other role does this mineral have in the body?
30. Name the mineral that is a component of several amino acids.
31. What type of diet pattern might be low in trace minerals? Why?
32. Identify the major role of iron in the body. Describe what happens when iron intake is inadequate.
33. Identify the mineral that is missing in the diet of someone with a goiter. Why is the lack of this mineral not as much of a problem today?
34. What foods are rich sources of copper?
35. Describe the relationship between fluoride and tooth decay. What is the usual source of fluoride?
36. What do scientists currently know about the role of zinc in human nutrition? Name several sources of zinc.

# 5 NUTRITIOUS FOODS FROM SOUP TO NUTS

With a noisy beep and a flashing cursor, Jenny's computer diet analysis signaled a low nutrient intake. The nutrient profile printout included the following message: "To stay healthy please consume 18 milligrams of iron and 60 milligrams of vitamin C each day." What foods should she choose to meet her iron and vitamin C needs?

Unemployment has forced George to change his life-style. Buying food on a limited budget is a new challenge. What foods provide similar nutrients but cost less?

Toia will be working at a summer youth camp. Camp residents, under her guidance, will be planning the meals. How can she be certain their meals meet caloric and nutrient needs?

Jimmy is responsible for the care of his younger brothers and sisters after school. The youngsters are always hungry. What snacks can he prepare that are fun and healthful?

Will you need to use the Recommended Daily Allowance (RDA) chart and a food composition table to answer these questions? No, there is an easier way: Following a food guide takes the hassle out of meal planning and diet evaluation.

*Your objectives in this chapter will be to:*

- *Use a food guide to assess diet adequacy*
- *List the dietary guidelines*
- *Compare the nutrient density of foods*
- *Use nutrition labeling to evaluate food products*
- *Plan nutritious meals and snacks*
- *Develop menus for different food budgets*

# BUILDING AN ADEQUATE DIET

For more than 65 years nutritionists and home economists have used food guides to assist consumers in selecting an adequate diet. Food guides are charts that group together foods of similar nutrient value. Specific information about portion size and number of daily servings from each group is included. This information translates nutrient needs into food. After all, people eat food, not nutrients. Using a food guide is a practical way to build an adequate diet.

As nutrition scientists gain more understanding of nutrient needs and balance, the RDAs are reevaluated. Food guides must also be updated to reflect new knowledge. In designing a food guide, nutritionists consider foods available, relative cost, and current food consumption patterns. In addition, a guide may emphasize certain foods. Foods highlighted may contain nutrients shown to be inadequate in recent nutritional surveys of the population.

The Hassle-Free Guide to a Better Diet is a revision of the Daily Food Guide (more commonly known as the "Basic Four") developed in the mid-1950s by the United States Department of

## THE HASSLE-FREE GUIDE TO A BETTER DIET

### Vegetable and Fruit Group

Have citrus fruit, melon, berries, or tomatoes daily and a dark-green or dark-yellow vegetable frequently. For a good source of fiber, eat unpeeled fruits and vegetables and fruits with edible seeds—berries or grapes. Choose 4 servings a day. One serving is:

| | | |
|---|---|---|
| ½ cup Vegetables | 1 medium-sized Potato | ½ Cantaloupe |
| 1 small Salad | 1 Orange | ½ Grapefruit |

*(Continued)*

Source: "The Hassle-Free Guide to a Better Diet," United States Department of Agriculture (Washington, D.C.: United States Government Printing Office, 1980), Leaflet No. 567.

### Bread and Cereal Group

Choose whole-grain products often. Choose 4 servings a day. One serving is:

| 1 slice Bread | ½ to ¾ cup cooked Cereal or Pasta | 1 oz Ready-to-Eat Cereal |
|---|---|---|

### Milk and Cheese Group

Skim, nonfat, and lowfat milk and milk products provide calcium and keep fat intake down. Choose 2 to 4 servings a day, as follows: adults, 2; children under 9 years old, 2-3; children 9 to 12 years old and pregnant women, 3; and teens and nursing mothers, 4.

| 1 cup Milk or Yogurt | 2 oz Processed Cheese Food | 2 cups Cottage Cheese |
|---|---|---|
| 1⅓ oz Cheddar or Swiss Cheese | 1½ cups Ice Cream or Ice Milk | |

### Meat, Fish, Poultry, and Beans Group

Poultry and fish have less fat content than red meats. Choose 2 servings a day. One serving is:

| 1 to 1½ oz lean, boneless, cooked Meat, Poultry, or Fish | ½ to ¾ cup cooked Dry Beans, Peas, Lentils, or Soybeans | ¼ to ½ cup Nuts, Sesame or Sunflower Seeds |
|---|---|---|
| 1 Egg | 2 tblsp Peanut Butter | |

### Fats, Sweets, and Alcohol Group

*CAUTION!* These foods provide calories but few nutrients.

**Table 5.1   Planning Breakfast Trade-offs with Similar Calories**

| Breakfast A | | Breakfast B | |
|---|---|---|---|
| **Food Item** | **Exchange Calories** | **Food Item** | **Exchange Calories** |
| ½ Grapefruit ......... | 40 | 4 Ounces Orange | |
| 1 Poached Egg ....... | 77.5 | Juice .............. | 40 |
| 1 Slice Whole | | 2 Tblsp Peanut | |
| Wheat Toast ....... | 70 | Butter ............ | 167.5 |
| 1 Cup Skim Milk .... | 80 | ½ English Muffin .. | 70 |
| Total Calories ..... | 267.5 | Total Calories .... | 277.5 |

Agriculture (USDA). The Daily Food Guide separated foods into four groups: Milk and Milk Products, Meat and Meat Alternates, Fruit and Vegetables, and Breads and Cereals. The revised Guide, presented on pages 108 and 109, divides foods into five groups based on their nutrient contribution. The major change is the addition of the fifth group of foods, which provide mainly Calories and few, if any, nutrients. Approximately 1200 Calories are provided by eating the minimum number of suggested servings from each group. Additional foods may be chosen from these groups to meet *your* calorie needs.

## Exchange System

Foods may also be placed in groups of equal energy value per specified serving size. The exchange system was designed in the 1950s for use by persons with diabetes mellitus. It was revised in 1976, stressing foods of lower cholesterol and fat content as the exchange base (refer to the Special Feature). For example, *skim milk* is the basis of one milk exchange. One milk exchange provides 8 grams of protein and 12 grams of carbohydrate, for a total of 80 Calories. If a milk product with a higher fat content is used, a fat exchange must be borrowed and omitted from the day's allotment. Each of the six exchange lists contains foods of similar energy and nutrient content. The carbohydrate, fat, protein, and energy values are indicated for each exchange. Serving sizes are adjusted to keep Calorie values equal. Think of the exchange system as similar to the different coins that can be combined to equal a dollar. See Table 5.1.

*Text continued on page 118.*

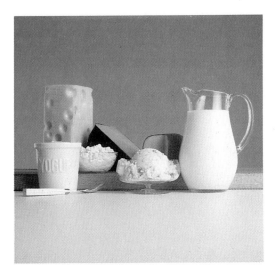

***Figure 5.1.*** Milk and milk products group.

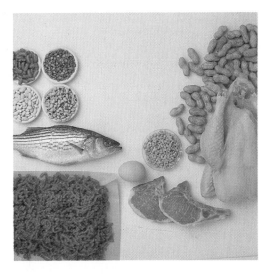

***Figure 5.2.*** Meat and meat alternates group.

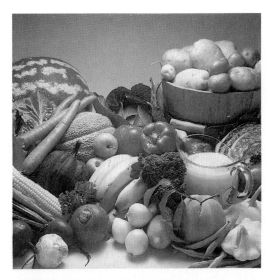

***Figure 5.3.*** Fruits and vegetables group.

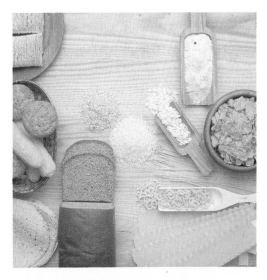

***Figure 5.4.*** Breads and cereals group.

# THE EXCHANGE SYSTEM

## Milk Exchanges

One exchange of milk contains 12 grams of carbohydrate, 8 grams of protein, a trace of fat, and 80 Calories. This list shows the kinds and amounts of milk or milk products to use for one Milk exchange. Those which appear in **bold type** are **nonfat**. Low-Fat and whole milk contain saturated fat.

**Non-Fat Fortified Milk**

**Skim or Non-Fat Milk** ............1 cup
**Powdered (Non-Fat Dry, before adding liquid)** ....................⅓ cup
**Canned, evaporated—Skim Milk** ................................½ cup
**Buttermilk made from Skim Milk** ................................1 cup
**Yogurt made from Skim Milk (plain, unflavored)** ..............1 cup

*Low-Fat Fortified Milk*

1% Fat Fortified milk (omit ½ Fat exchange) ..........................1 cup

*Low-Fat Fortified Milk (cont'd )*

2% Fat Fortified milk (omit 1 Fat exchange) ..........................1 cup
Yogurt made from 2% fortified milk (plain, unflavored)  (omit 1 Fat exchange) ...................1 cup

*Whole Milk (Omit 2 Fat exchanges)*

Whole Milk ...........................1 cup
Canned, evaporated Whole Milk ..½ cup
Buttermilk made from Whole Milk ................................1 cup
Yogurt made from Whole Milk (plain, unflavored) ................1 cup

## Vegetable Exchanges

One exchange of vegetables contains about 5 grams of carbohydrate, 2 grams of protein, and 25 Calories. This list shows the kinds of vegetables to use for one vegetable exchange. One exchange is ½ cup.

Source: The exchange lists from the "Exchange Lists for Meal Planning" were prepared by committees of the American Diabetes Association, Inc., and The American Dietetic Association in cooperation with the National Institute of Arthritis, Metabolism and Digestive Diseases and the National Heart and Lung Institute, National Institutes of Health, Public Health Service, U.S. Department of Health, Education and Welfare. Copyright American Diabetes Association, Inc., The American Dietetic Association, 1976.

| | | | |
|---|---|---|---|
| Asparagus | Eggplant | Greens: | String Beans, |
| Bean Sprouts | Green Pepper | Spinach | green or yellow |
| Beets | Greens: | Turnip | Summer Squash |
| Broccoli | Beet | Mushrooms | Tomatoes |
| Brussels Sprouts | Chards | Okra | Tomato Juice |
| Cabbage | Collards | Onions | Turnips |
| Carrots | Dandelion | Rhubarb | Vegetable Juice |
| Cauliflower | Kale | Rutabaga | Cocktail |
| Celery | Mustard | Sauerkraut | Zucchini |
| Cucumbers | | | |

The following raw vegetables may be used as desired:

| | | | |
|---|---|---|---|
| Chicory | Endive | Lettuce | Radishes |
| Chinese Cabbage | Escarole | Parsley | Watercress |

Starchy Vegetables are found in the Bread Exchange List.

## Fruit Exchange

One exchange of fruit contains 10 grams of carbohydrate and 40 Calories. This list shows the kinds and amounts of fruits to use for one fruit exchange.

| | | | |
|---|---|---|---|
| Apple | 1 small | Grapefruit | ½ |
| Apple Juice | ⅓ cup | Grapefruit Juice | ½ cup |
| Applesauce (unsweetened) | ½ cup | Grapes | 12 |
| Apricots, fresh | 2 medium | Grape Juice | ¼ cup |
| Apricots, dried | 4 halves | Mango | ½ small |
| Banana | ½ small | Melon | |
| Berries | | Cantaloupe | ¼ small |
| Blackberries | ½ cup | Honeydew | ⅛ medium |
| Blueberries | ½ cup | Watermelon | 1 cup |
| Raspberries | ½ cup | Nectarine | 1 small |
| Strawberries | ¾ cup | Orange | 1 small |
| Cherries | 10 large | Orange Juice | ½ cup |
| Cider | ⅓ cup | Papaya | ¾ cup |
| Dates | 2 | Peach | 1 medium |
| Figs, fresh | 1 | Pear | 1 small |
| Figs, dried | 1 | Persimmon, native | 1 medium |

*(Continued)*

## THE EXCHANGE SYSTEM (cont'd)

| | |
|---|---|
| Pineapple .......................½ cup | Prune Juice ......................¼ cup |
| Pineapple Juice ................⅓ cup | Raisins ...........................2 tblsp |
| Plums ...........................2 medium | Tangerine .......................1 medium |
| Prunes...........................2 medium | |

Cranberries may be used as desired if no sugar is added.

### Bread Exchanges (includes Bread, Cereal, and Starchy Vegetables)

One exchange of bread contains 15 grams of carbohydrate, 2 grams of protein, and 70 Calories. This list shows the kinds and amounts of breads, cereals, starchy vegetables, and prepared foods to use for one bread exchange. Those which appear in **bold type** are **low-fat.**

### Bread

**White (including French and**
  **Italian)**............................1 slice
**Whole Wheat**......................1 slice
**Rye or Pumpernickel**...........1 slice
**Raisin** .............................1 slice
**Bagel, small** .....................½
**English Muffin, small** ..........½
**Plain Roll, bread** ...............1
**Frankfurter Roll**.................½
**Hamburger Bun** .................½
**Dried Bread Crumbs** ...........3 tblsp
**Tortilla, 6″**........................1

### Cereal

**Bran Flakes**......................½ cup
**Other Ready-to-Eat**
  **unsweetened Cereal**..........¾ cup
**Puffed Cereal**
  **(unfrosted)** .....................1 cup

### Cereal (cont'd)

**Cereal (cooked)** ..................½ cup
**Grits (cooked)** ....................½ cup
**Rice or Barley (cooked)** ........½ cup
**Pasta (cooked), Spaghetti,**
  **Noodles, Macaroni**...........½ cup
**Popcorn (popped, no fat**
  **added)** ..........................3 cups
**Cornmeal (dry)** .................2 tblsp
**Flour** ..............................2½
  tblsp
**Wheat Germ** .....................¼ cup

### Crackers

**Arrowroot** .......................3
**Graham, 2½″**.....................2
**Matzoth, 4″ x 6″**.................½
**Oyster**.............................20
**Pretzels** ..........................25
**Rye Wafers, 2″ x 3½″** ..........3

**Saltines** ...........................6
**Soda, 2½″** ........................4

**Dried Beans, Peas, and Lentils**
  **Beans, Peas, Lentils**
    **(dried and cooked)** ...........½ cup
  **Baked Beans, no Pork**
    **(canned)** ........................¼ cup

**Starchy Vegetables**
  **Corn**................................⅓ cup
  **Corn on the Cob**.................1 small
  **Lima Beans**......................½ cup
  **Parsnips** ...........................2/3 cup
  **Peas, Green (canned**
    **or frozen)** .....................½ cup
  **Potato, White** ...................1 small
  **Potato (mashed)** ................½ cup
  **Pumpkin** ........................¾ cup
  **Winter Squash, Acorn**
    **or Butternut**..................½ cup
  **Yam or Sweet Potato**...........¼ cup

Prepared Foods

Biscuit, 2″ .........................1
  (omit 1 Fat exchange)
Corn Bread, 2″ x 2″ x 1″ ........1
  (omit 1 Fat exchange)
Corn Muffin, 2″..................1
  (omit 1 Fat exchange)
Crackers, round butter ..........5
  (omit 1 Fat exchange)
Muffin, plain small ...............1
  (omit 1 Fat exchange)
Potatoes, French Fried,
  length 2″ to 3½″...............8
  (omit 1 Fat exchange)
Potato or Corn Chips ............15
  (omit 2 Fat exchanges)
Pancake, 5″ x ½″.................1
  (omit 1 Fat exchange)
Waffle, 5″ x ½″...................1
  (omit 1 Fat exchange)

## Meat Exchanges

One exchange of lean meat (1 oz) contains 7 grams of protein, 3 grams of fat, and 55 Calories.

This list shows the kinds and amounts of lean meat and other protein-rich foods to use for one low-fat meat exchange.

Beef:    Baby Beef (very lean), Chipped Beef, Chuck, Flank Steak, Tenderloin, Plate Ribs, Plate Skirt Steak, Round (bottom, top), All cuts Rump, Spare Ribs, and Tripe.....................1 oz

Lamb:   Leg, Rib, Sirloin, Loin (Roast and Chops), Shank, and Shoulder................................................................1 oz

Pork:    Leg (Whole Rump, Center Shank), Ham, and Smoked (center slices)...........................................................................1 oz

*(Continued)*

## THE EXCHANGE SYSTEM (cont'd)

Veal:      Leg, Loin, Rib, Shank, Shoulder, and Cutlets .....................1 oz
Poultry:   Meat without skin of Chicken, Turkey, Cornish Hen, Guinea
           Hen, and Pheasant ...................................................1 oz
Fish:      Any fresh or frozen ......................................................1 oz
           Canned Salmon, Tuna, Mackerel, Crab and Lobster,.............¼ cup
           Clams, Oysters, Scallops, Shrimp, and ..........................5 or 1 oz
           Sardines, drained ......................................................3
Cheeses containing less than 5% Butterfat ......................................1 oz
Cottage Cheese, Dry and 2% Butterfat ...........................................¼ cup
Dried Beans and Peas (omit 1 Bread exchange)................................½ cup

### For one exchange of Medium-Fat Meat (1 oz), omit ½ Fat exchange.

This list shows the kinds and amounts of medium-fat meat and other protein-rich foods to use for one medium-fat meat exchange.

Beef:     Ground (15% fat), Corned Beef (canned), Rib Eye, and Round
          (ground commercial) .................................................1 oz
Pork:     Loin (all cuts Tenderloin), Shoulder Arm (picnic), Shoulder
          Blade, Boston Butt, Canadian Bacon, and Boiled Ham .......1 oz
Liver, Heart, Kidney, and Sweetbreads (these are high in cholesterol) ......1 oz
Cottage Cheese, creamed ........................................................¼ cup
Cheese:   Mozzarella, Ricotta, Farmer's cheese, Neufchatel, and...........1 oz
          Parmesan .............................................................3 tblsp
Egg (high in cholesterol)........................................................1
**Peanut Butter** (omit 2 additional Fat exchanges)..............................2 tblsp

### For one exchange of High-Fat Meat (1 oz), omit ½ Fat exchange.

This list shows the kinds and amounts of high-fat meat and other protein-rich foods to use for one high-fat meat exchange.

Beef:     Brisket, Corned Beef (Brisket), Ground Beef (more than 20%
          fat), Hamburger (commercial), Chuck (ground commercial),
          Roasts (Rib), and Steaks (Club and Rib) .........................1 oz

| | | |
|---|---|---|
| Lamb: | Breast | 1 oz |
| Pork: | Spare Ribs, Loin (Back Ribs), Pork (ground), Country style Ham, and Deviled Ham | 1 oz |
| Veal: | Breast | 1 oz |
| Poultry: | Capon, Duck (domestic), Goose | 1 oz |
| Cheese: | Cheddar Types | 1 oz |
| Cold Cuts | | 4½" x ⅛" slice |
| Frankfurter | | 1 small |

## Fat Exchanges

One exchange of Fat contains 5 grams of fat and 45 Calories. This list shows the kinds and amounts of fat-containing foods to use for one fat exchange. To plan a diet low in saturated fat, select only those exchanges that appear in **bold type.** They are **polyunsaturated.**

| | | | |
|---|---|---|---|
| **Margarine, soft, tub or stick**[a] | 1 tsp | Margarine, regular stick | 1 tsp |
| **Avocado (4″ diameter)**[b] | ⅛ | Butter | 1 tsp |
| **Oil, Corn, Cottonseed, Safflower, Soy, and Sunflower** | 1 tsp | Bacon fat | 1 tsp |
| | | Bacon, crisp | 1 strip |
| | | Cream, light | 2 tblsp |
| **Oil, Olive**[b] | 1 tsp | Cream, Sour | 2 tblsp |
| **Oil, Peanut**[b] | 1 tsp | Cream, heavy | 1 tblsp |
| **Olives**[b] | 5 small | Cream Cheese | 1 tblsp |
| **Almonds**[b] | 10 whole | French Dressing[c] | 1 tblsp |
| **Pecans**[b] | 2 large whole | Italian Dressing[c] | 1 tblsp |
| **Peanuts**[b] | | Lard | 1 tsp |
| **Spanish** | 20 whole | Mayonnaise[c] | 1 tsp |
| **Virginia** | 10 whole | Salad Dressing, Mayonnaise type[c] | 2 tsp |
| **Walnuts** | 6 small | Salt Pork | ¾" cube |
| **Nuts, other**[b] | 6 small | | |

[a]Made with corn, cottonseed, safflower, soy, or sunflower oil only.
[b]Fat content is primarily monounsaturated.
[c]If made with corn, cottonseed, safflower, soy, or sunflower oil, can be used on fat-modified diet.

Weight control diets may be planned using the exchange system. First, a desirable Calorie level for weight loss must be determined. Next, food preferences and nutrient needs must be considered in allocating exchanges to meet the Calorie level. The diet plan indicates the number of exchanges allowed each day from each group. This permits individuals to choose freely the foods they prefer without counting Calories. However, *only* the indicated portion size can be consumed. More information on weight control will be covered in Chapter 7.

## Dietary Guidelines

For many Americans, obtaining enough food for an adequate diet is not a problem. However, some dietary practices may be related to the development of chronic disease. Practices associated with an increased chance of disease are called *risk factors.* For example, eating too much often leads to *obesity,* or an excess of body fat. This topic will be covered in depth in Chapter 7. The Surgeon General of the United States warns that obesity is clearly related to diabetes, gallbladder disease, and high blood pressure. It may also contribute to heart disease, arthritis, gout, and respiratory disease. Thus not only is obesity itself a problem, it is also a risk factor for several other diseases.

Scientific debate continues over the precise relationship between diet and disease. Until this relationship is defined, what advice

---

### Table 5.2   Dietary Guidelines for Americans

1. Eat a variety of foods
2. Maintain desirable weight
3. Avoid too much fat, saturated fat, and cholesterol
4. Eat foods with adequate starch and fiber
5. Avoid too much sugar
6. Avoid too much sodium
7. If you drink alcoholic beverages, do so in moderation

Source: United States Department of Agriculture and United States Department of Health and Human Services, "Nutrition and Your Health: Dietary Guidelines for Americans" (Washington, D.C.: United States Government Printing Office, 1985).

should Americans follow? Based on current knowledge, dietary moderation and nutrient balance are safe and healthy objectives. Nutritionists in the federal government have developed a set of guidelines to assist consumers in achieving these objectives. *Nutrition and Your Health: Dietary Guidelines for Americans* is a joint publication of the Department of Health and Human Services and the USDA. See Table 5.2.

The issues surrounding the diet and health controversy are covered in Chapter 6. Suggestions for applying these guidelines are also discussed.

# COMPARING FOODS FOR NUTRIENT VALUE

Foods within any food group or exchange vary in actual nutrient value. For example, not all green vegetables are equally good sources of vitamin A. One-half cup of green beans provides 330 I.U. (international units) of vitamin A, while a similar portion of broccoli contains 1970 I.U. Pears and apples are poor sources of vitamin C, but strawberries, cantaloupe, or citrus fruits, such as oranges and grapefruit, are excellent sources of vitamin C. Being aware of this variation helps a person make better choices within food groups or exchanges. Selecting a variety of foods from each group or exchange each day is a good way to obtain needed nutrients.

## Effects of Processing

In addition to natural nutrient variation, processing may alter a food's nutrient content. For example, the milling of cereal grains removes important vitamins and minerals. Processors may *enrich* their products with several of the lost nutrients. Nutrients frequently added back to processed foods are thiamin, riboflavin, niacin, and iron. However, various trace minerals and fiber will still be missing. See Table 5.3. Compare the nutrient content of a loaf of enriched white bread and a loaf of whole wheat bread. What nutrients have been added back to the white bread? Chapter 10 will discuss this subject further.

### Table 5.3   Selected Nutrient Content of Bread

| 1 Loaf of Bread | Thiamin (mg) | Riboflavin (mg) | Niacin (mg) | Iron (mg) |
|---|---|---|---|---|
| White unenriched with 3% to 4% Non-Fat Dry Milk...................... | 0.31 | 0.39 | 5.0 | 3.2 |
| White enriched with 3% to 4% Non-Fat Dry Milk...................... | 1.8 | 1.1 | 15.0 | 11.3 |
| Whole Wheat made with 2% Non-Fat Dry Milk...................... | 1.17 | 0.56 | 12.9 | 10.4 |

Source: United States Department of Health, Education, and Welfare and the Food and Drug Administration, "Standard of Identity for Bakery Products," *Federal Register* 36 (1971):23074, 38 (1973):28558, and 39 (1974):5188.

### Effects of Preparation

The method of preparation also alters nutrient and caloric content. See Table 5.4. Compare the nutrient and Calorie differences between a baked potato, french fries, and potato chips. Now, what happens to the caloric value when you add sour cream, butter, and bacon bits to the baked potato? Consumers must consider these differences in food value.

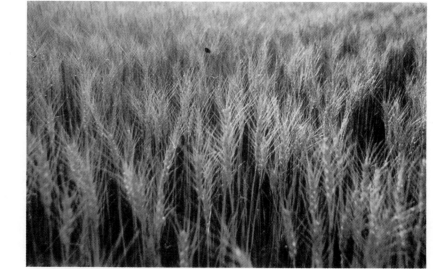

*Figure 5.5.*  The milling of cereal grains removes important vitamins and minerals.

## Table 5.4    Different Forms of Potatoes

|  | Calories | Ascorbic Acid (mg) |
|---|---|---|
| ½ Medium Baked Potato............ | 73 | 15 |
| 10 French Fried Strips .............. | 110 | 11 |
| 10 Potato Chips ...................... | 115 | 3 |

Source: United Stated Department of Agriculture, "Nutritive Value of Foods" (Washington, D.C.: United States Government Printing Office, 1981), Home and Garden Bulletin No. 72.

Some of the common changes during preparation are in food shape and texture. Foods may be chopped, diced, sliced, mashed, cooked, or frozen. Flavor, spices, and sauces are often added during preparation.

The method of food preparation is influenced by cultural background, health values, attitudes about food use, available equipment, economic status, and personal preference. Some frequently used methods are broiling, boiling, steaming, baking, and frying. See Table 5.5. Adding fats, such as margarine, butter, lard, or oil, to food during preparation can quickly raise its caloric value. Because fat

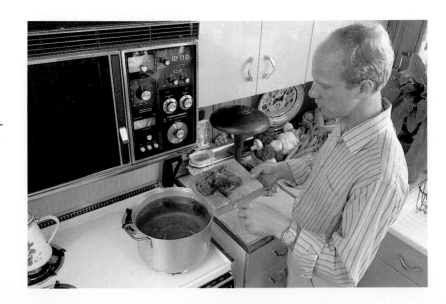

*Figure 5.6.* Water-soluble vitamins are lost by overcooking vegetables in too much water.

## Table 5.5    Methods of Food Preparation

| Method | Equipment/Procedure | Type of Heat |
|---|---|---|
| Broiling | Rack or spit exposed to open flame | Dry |
| Pan Broiling | Electric skillet or fry pan with no added moisture or fat | Dry |
| Pan Frying or Stir Frying | Fry pan, electric skillet, or wok to which a small amount of fat is added | Dry |
| Deep-Fat Frying | Sauce pan or deep fryer to which enough fat is added to submerge food | Dry |
| Baking or Roasting | Oven, covered grill, or oven-like appliance | Dry |
| Boiling or Stewing | Pot or pan to which liquid has been added and heated to boiling point | Moist |
| Steaming | A pan of boiling water with a basket to hold food above the water. Pressure cooking is a variation | Moist |
| Simmering or Slow Cooking | Pot, pan, or slow cooker in which food and liquid are allowed to simmer for a long time | Moist |
| Microwaving | Microwave oven in which the magnetron tube generates microwaves, causing water molecules to vibrate and heat food | None |

contributes 9 Calories per gram (one teaspoon equals 5 grams), a teaspoon of butter adds an extra 45 Calories. Food processing will be discussed in more detail in Chapter 10.

## Effects of Storage

How food is stored influences food quality. Food scientists

have studied the effects of different storage on the nutrient content, taste, appearance, and safety of food. For example, a potato stored at temperatures below 40° F will become sweeter because the starch is changed to sugar. Cutting a grapefruit and leaving the cut half exposed to air will result in loss of vitamin C. To avoid this loss, cut citrus fruits just before serving or cover with plastic wrap after cutting. Also, prepare only the amount of orange juice you will use within a day or two, because prolonged exposure to air will decrease the vitamin C content.

## Nutrient Density

What is a nutritious food? Orange juice is more nutritious than a soft drink because nutritional quality is simply a function of a food's nutrient content. However, being nutritious is also related to the number of Calories provided by a food. What quantity of a nutrient is provided per Calorie? What proportion of a person's nutrient and Calorie allowance is met by the food?

The nutritional value of food can be determined by a mathematical formula to determine a percentage. The formula is referred to as the *Index of Nutritional Quality* (INQ). This formula is:

$$INQ = \frac{\text{Amount of nutrient/Calorie content of food}}{\text{Allowance for nutrient/Calorie allowance}}$$

An INQ of 1 or more means that a food has a positive nutrient/energy ratio. In other words, the food is *nutrient dense*. See Table 5.6. The nutrient density of a food may also be visually represented by a bar graph. The nutritional quality of a food item or meal may be assessed

### Table 5.6    Calculating Nutritional Quality

One Slice Whole Wheat Bread contains 3 gm Protein and 65 Calories.

An 18-year-old Woman needs:
46 gm Protein/Day
2100 Calories/Day

$$\frac{\text{Protein}}{\text{Calories}} = \frac{3/46}{65/2100} = 2:1$$

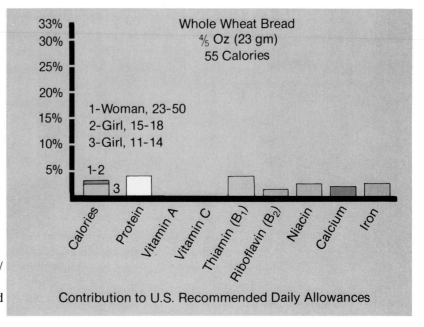

*Illustration 5.1.*
Comparison of Nutrient/
Calorie Contents for
Whole Wheat Bread and
Danish Pastry Roll.
Adapted from the Na-
tional Dairy Council
Publication B043 (Chi-
cago, Ill.: National
Dairy Council, 1974).
Courtesy Comparison
Cards, National Dairy
Council.

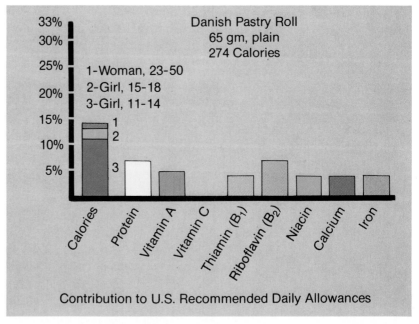

by comparing the length of the nutrient bar to that of the energy bar. See Illustration 5.1.

### Nutrition Labeling

How does a consumer judge the nutritional value of a commercially processed food or an imitation product? In response to consumer demand, food manufacturers agreed to print nutrient information on food product labels. However, a list of nutrients contained in the product is meaningless without a standard of reference. For example, what does it mean if a 16 ounce can of beef stew contains 24 grams of protein?

It would be nice to know the amount of a nutrient provided by a single serving of the item as compared to your personal RDA for that nutrient. However, that is not practical because RDA levels vary. There just isn't space on a label for all the RDA age and sex categories. Therefore, the Food and Drug Administration (FDA) designed the *United States Recommended Daily Allowances* (U.S. RDAs) for use in nutrition labeling. See Table 5.7. The U.S. RDA represents the highest allowance from the 1968 RDA for eight major nutrients: protein, vitamin A, vitamin C, thiamin, riboflavin, niacin, calcium, and iron. Thus an intake of 100% of the U.S. RDA meets or exceeds a person's RDA.

By law, nutrition information must appear on labels of all fortified foods and all foods for which a nutrition claim is made. Food product labels must indicate the percentage of the U.S. RDA contained per serving for these nutrients. Other nutrients, such as sodium, may be listed. In addition, the label must show the number of servings per container and list the grams of carbohydrate, protein, and fat. For ease of comparison, a uniform format for a nutrition label is required. See Table 5.8. Chapter 10 will take a closer look at what is in the package.

## PLANNING MEALS AND SNACKS

Are your food choices planned, or do they just happen? Are regular meals or eating times a part of your daily schedule? Frequently individual and family activities shape meal patterns. Today an

**Table 5.7     U.S. Recommended Daily Allowances (U.S. RDA)**

Protein
    Protein quality equal to or greater
        than casein............................45 gm
    Protein quality less than casein.......65 gm
Vitamin A ..................................5,000 International Units
Vitamin C (ascorbic acid)................60 mg
Thiamin (vitamin $B_1$) ....................1.5 mg
Riboflavin (vitamin $B_2$)...................1.7 mg
Niacin ......................................20 mg
Calcium......................................1.0 gram
Iron..........................................18 mg
Vitamin D ..................................400 International Units
Vitamin E...................................30 International Units
Vitamin $B_6$ ..............................2.0 mg
Folic acid (folacin) ........................0.4 mg
Vitamin $B_{12}$ ..............................6 μg
Phosphorus ................................1.0 gm
Iodine ......................................150 μg
Magnesium..................................400 mg
Zinc ........................................15 mg
Copper .....................................2 mg
Biotin ......................................0.3 mg
Pantothenic acid ...........................10 mg

Source: Food and Drug Administration, "We Want You to Know What We Know About Nutrition Labels on Food" (Washington, D.C.: United States Government Printing Office, 1973), Department of Health and Human Services Publication No. (FDA) 73-2039.

increasing number of meals and snacks are eaten away from home. Food advertising encourages impulse or unplanned eating. An advertisement can be so powerful as to trigger a person to interrupt activity for a "food break." Personal reactions to emotional stress and boredom may also prompt impulse eating. Haphazard food selection often causes nutritional imbalance. In addition, it is usually more costly. Planning is the key to nutritious, economical eating.

| Table 5.8 | Minimum Information Required on a Nutrition Label |
|---|---|

Nutrition Information
(Per Serving)
Serving Size = 1 oz
Servings Per Container = 12

Calories ..............................110
Protein ................................2 grams
Carbohydrate .......................24 grams
Fat .....................................0 gram

Percentage of U.S. Recommended Daily
Allowances (U.S. RDA)[a]

Protein..........................................2
Thiamin .......................................8
Niacin .........................................2

[a]Contains less than 2% of U.S. RDA for vitamin A, vitamin C, riboflavin, calcium, and iron.

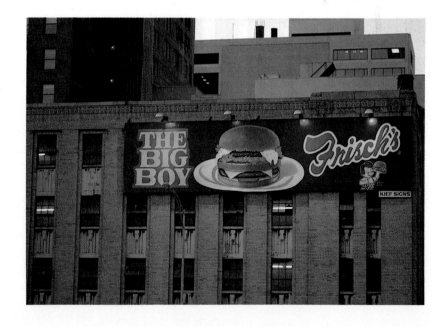

***Figure 5.7.*** Food advertisements can trigger impulse buying and eating.

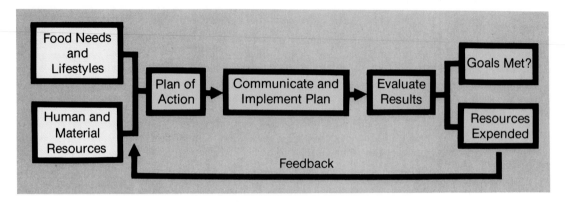

***Illustration 5.2.***    Food Management Decision-Making Process.

Whether you live on your own or share household responsibilities, providing appealing, nutritious, and economical meals is a challenge. The process of food management includes meal planning, food purchasing and storage, and meal preparation and service. Food management for the beginner may be frustrating and time consuming. The tasks can be made easier and more rewarding by considering the forces that influence the decision-making process. See Illustration 5.2.

## Determine a Plan of Action

***Goals and Resources.*** First, determine your meal pattern needs while considering the members of your household and their life-styles. Ask such questions as:
- How many and which meals will be eaten at home?
- What type of meal pattern fits your life-style?
- What are the nutritional needs of members of your household?
- What are the individual food preferences or special requirements?
- How much money is available to spend on food each week or month?
- Who will be responsible for various food management tasks, including shopping, meal preparation, and clean-up?
- What kitchen equipment is available for food storage, preparation, and service?

After assessing your household, consider the food preparer's knowledge and skills. Regardless of his or her level of expertise, a cookbook is essential. Acquire a comprehensive cookbook that provides tested recipes for all the foods needed for a healthful diet, "from soup to nuts." You can expand your cookbook selection as your interests and needs dictate. It will also be necessary to identify a general schedule for shopping and preparation. Obviously, a meal cannot be prepared if the refrigerator and cupboards are empty!

***Managing Your Food Budget.*** The most difficult task in food management is defining and staying within a food budget. This decision should be made before meals are planned and must be considered in making necessary food substitutions during shopping. Individuals and families have different amounts of money available to meet their everyday needs. Thus the USDA developed food plans to assist consumers in planning nutritious meals at different levels of cost: thrifty, low, moderate, and liberal. Current food prices, eating patterns, and new data on food composition were considered. Moreover, an allowance was made for food waste. Table 5.9 shows the estimated cost to purchase food based on each of these plans according to families and age groups for a child, a male, and a female.

Table 5.10 shows the amount of food to be served daily for

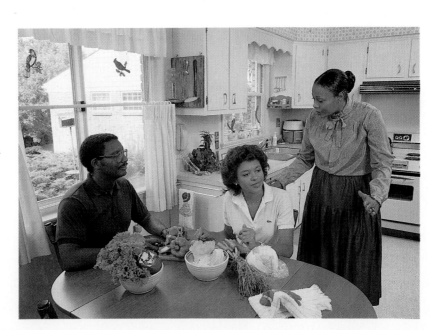

***Figure 5.8.*** Managing food for a household requires input and cooperation from everyone.

## Table 5.9   Compare Food Plan Costs[a]

| | Cost for 1 week ($) | | | | Cost for 1 month ($) | | | |
|---|---|---|---|---|---|---|---|---|
| | Thrifty Plan | Low-cost Plan | Moderate-Cost Plan | Liberal Plan | Thrifty Plan | Low-cost Plan | Moderate-Cost Plan | Liberal Plan |
| **Families** | | | | | | | | |
| Family of 2[b] | | | | | | | | |
| 20-50 years.......... | 37.50 | 47.20 | 58.10 | 71.70 | 162.50 | 204.30 | 251.60 | 310.70 |
| 51 years and over.... | 35.50 | 45.10 | 55.40 | 66.10 | 153.70 | 195.40 | 240.40 | 286.50 |
| Family of 4 | | | | | | | | |
| Couple, 20-50 years and children | | | | | | | | |
| 1-2 and 3-5 years | 54.50 | 67.70 | 82.60 | 100.90 | 236.00 | 293.50 | 357.90 | 437.30 |
| 6-8 and 9-11 years.......... | 62.60 | 79.70 | 99.40 | 119.40 | 271.10 | 345.20 | 430.90 | 517.40 |
| **Individuals[c]** | | | | | | | | |
| Child | | | | | | | | |
| 1-2 years.......... | 9.80 | 11.80 | 13.80 | 16.50 | 42.40 | 51.30 | 59.70 | 71.60 |
| 3-5 years.......... | 10.60 | 13.00 | 16.00 | 19.20 | 45.90 | 56.50 | 69.50 | 83.20 |
| 6-8 years.......... | 13.00 | 17.20 | 21.50 | 25.10 | 56.40 | 74.60 | 93.30 | 108.90 |
| 9-11 years.......... | 15.50 | 19.60 | 25.10 | 29.10 | 67.00 | 84.90 | 108.90 | 126.00 |
| Male | | | | | | | | |
| 12-14 years.......... | 16.20 | 22.20 | 27.70 | 32.50 | 70.20 | 96.30 | 119.90 | 140.60 |
| 15-19 years.......... | 16.80 | 23.10 | 28.50 | 33.00 | 73.00 | 100.00 | 123.50 | 143.10 |
| 20-50 years.......... | 17.90 | 22.80 | 28.50 | 34.30 | 77.60 | 98.80 | 123.50 | 148.50 |
| 51 years and over.... | 16.30 | 21.60 | 26.50 | 31.70 | 70.50 | 93.60 | 114.90 | 137.40 |
| Female | | | | | | | | |
| 12-19 years.......... | 16.10 | 19.30 | 23.30 | 28.10 | 69.70 | 83.40 | 100.90 | 121.60 |
| 20-50 years.......... | 16.20 | 20.10 | 24.30 | 30.90 | 70.10 | 86.90 | 105.20 | 134.00 |
| 51 years and over.... | 16.00 | 19.40 | 23.90 | 28.40 | 69.20 | 84.00 | 103.60 | 123.10 |

Source: United States Department of Agriculture (Hyattsville, Md.: United States Department of Agriculture, 1985). Human Nutrition Information Service Nutrition Education Division Hyattsville, Maryland 20782

[a]Cost of food at home estimated for food plans at four cost levels, February 1985, U.S. Average.

[b]Ten percent added for family size adjustment (see footnote c).

[c]The costs given are for individuals in four-person families. For individuals in other size families, the following adjustments are suggested: one-person—add 20%; two-person—add 10%; three-person—add 5%; five- or six-person—subtract 5%; seven- or more-person—subtract 10%.

each plan. The amount needed for each household member can be tallied. Then, the information can be used to plan meals or make a grocery list. As the budget increases, quantities of meat, fish, poultry, fruits, and vegetables increase. On the other hand, quantities of grain products and dried beans and peas decrease. Thus the thrifty plan includes larger amounts of foods that are economical nutrient sources. This plan is the basis for federal Food Stamp Program benefits. Sample meals and recipes to follow the thrifty plan are also available from the federal government.

## Communicate and Implement the Plan

*Menu Planning.* Assemble cookbooks, magazines, and newspapers that might provide meal and recipe ideas. Check the newspaper for grocery store specials and food coupons that might be of use. Planning meals for a week at a time assures food variety and efficiency in grocery shopping. It may be helpful to use a menu planning chart similar to the one in Table 5.11. First, identify the *entree,* or main dish, for each meal to be served during the week. Then fill in the fruits, vegetables, breads, cereals, milk products, and beverages that complement the entree. Desserts may be added if desired. As you select foods to complete each meal, consider the overall color, flavor, texture, and nutrient content. Avoid planning meals that contain foods of all the same flavor or color. Remember, eating should be an enjoyable experience! Next, check a food guide to make certain meals and snacks meet household members' daily nutrient needs. Today many people eat snacks, or minimeals, instead of three larger meals. Spend your food budget wisely and plan snacks that add nutrients as well as Calories.

*Inventory.* After meals and snacks are planned, take a quick inventory of the cupboards, refrigerator, and freezer for foods already on hand. Make certain the supply of staple items, such as flour, sugar, and spices, is adequate. Then prepare a grocery list of foods needed for the week. See Table 5.12. Indicate the size package or amount needed of each item. Also specify the form of the food needed, such as fresh, frozen, or canned. Buy the form that most closely meets your need. For example, canned pineapple is a more cost-effective choice than the fresh fruit when used in a gelatin salad.

## Table 5.10    Food Plans at Four Costs: Food to Serve Each Day[a]

| Food Plan and Family Member | Milk[b] (cup) | Cooked Lean Meat or Alternate[c] (oz) | Vegetables and Fruit[d] (½ cup) | Cereal and Bakery Products[e] (portion) |
|---|---|---|---|---|
| **Thrifty Plan** | | | | |
| Child | | | | |
| 1-5 years | 2 | 1½ to 2 | 2 | 3 or more |
| 6-11 years | 2 to 3 | 2½ to 3 | 2½ to 3½ | 6 or more |
| Male | | | | |
| 12-19 years | 3 | 3 to 4 | 3 to 4 | 7 or more |
| 20-54 years | 1½ | 4 to 5 | 3 to 4 | 7 or more |
| 55 years and over | 1½ | 4 | 3 to 4 | 7 or more |
| Female | | | | |
| 12-19 years | 3 | 3 | 3 to 4 | 5 or more |
| 20-54 years | 1½ | 4 | 3 to 4 | 5 or more |
| 55 years and over | 1½ | 3 | 3 to 4 | 5 or more |
| **Low-Cost Plan** | | | | |
| Child | | | | |
| 1-5 years | 2 to 3 | 2 to 3 | 2 to 3 | 3 or more |
| 6-11 years | 2 to 3 | 3 to 4 | 3 to 4 | 5 or more |
| Male | | | | |
| 12-19 years | 3 to 4 | 5 to 6 | 4 to 5 | 6 or more |
| 20-54 years | 1½ to 2 | 6 to 7 | 4 to 5 | 6 or more |
| 55 years and over | 1½ to 2 | 5 | 4 to 5 | 6 or more |

Source: United States Department of Agriculture, "Family Food Budgeting . . . For Good Meals and Good Nutrition (Washington, D.C.: United States Government Printing Office, 1981), Home and Garden Bulletin No. 94.

[a] Amounts shown allow for some plate waste.

[b] As alternates: ¾ oz of hard cheese or ¾ cup of cottage cheese, ice cream, or ice milk or ½ cup of unflavored yogurt may replace ½ cup of fluid milk.

[c] As alternates: 1 oz of cooked poultry or fish, one egg, ½ cup of cooked dry beans or peas, or 2 tablespoons of peanut butter may replace 1 oz of cooked lean meat.

[d] One-half cup of vegetable or fruit or a portion—one medium apple, banana, or half a medium grapefruit or cantaloup. Smaller portions may be served, especially to young children.

[e] A portion is two slices of bread, one hamburger bun, one large muffin or cup cake, 1 ounce ready-to-eat cereal, or ¾ cup cooked cereal, such as oatmeal, rice, spaghetti, macaroni, or noodles. Smaller servings may be given, especially to young children, girls, and women; but the total daily amounts on the average should add up to portions listed.

## Table 5.10 (cont'd)

| Food Plan and Family Member | Milk[b] (cup) | Cooked Lean Meat or Alternate[c] (oz) | Vegetables and Fruit[d] (½ cup) | Cereal and Bakery Products[e] (portion) |
|---|---|---|---|---|
| **Low-Cost Plan (cont'd)** | | | | |
| Female | | | | |
| 12-19 years | 3 to 4 | 4 | 4 | 5 or more |
| 20-54 years | 1½ to 2 | 4 to 5 | 4 | 5 or more |
| 55 years and over | 1½ to 2 | 3 to 4 | 4 | 5 or more |
| **Moderate-Cost Plan** | | | | |
| Child | | | | |
| 1-5 years | 2 to 3 | 2½ to 3 | 2 to 3 | 3 or more |
| 6-11 years | 3 to 4 | 4 to 5 | 4 to 5 | 4 or more |
| Male | | | | |
| 12-19 years | 4 | 5 to 7 | 4½ to 5½ | 6 or more |
| 20-54 years | 2 | 7 to 8 | 5 to 6 | 6 or more |
| 55 years and over | 2 | 6 to 7 | 5 to 6 | 5 or more |
| Female | | | | |
| 12-19 years | 3½ to 4 | 4 to 5 | 4 to 5 | 4 or more |
| 20-54 years | 2 | 5 to 6 | 4 to 5 | 4 or more |
| 55 years and over | 2 | 4 to 5 | 5 | 4 or more |
| **Liberal Plan** | | | | |
| Child | | | | |
| 1-5 years | 2½ to 3 | 3 to 3½ | 3 to 4 | 3 or more |
| 6-11 years | 3½ to 4½ | 5 to 6 | 5 to 6 | 4 or more |
| Male | | | | |
| 12-19 years | 4 to 4½ | 6 to 8 | 5 to 6 | 5 or more |
| 20-54 years | 2 | 9 | 6 to 7 | 5 or more |
| 55 years and over | 2 | 7 to 8 | 6 to 7 | 5 or more |
| Female | | | | |
| 12-19 years | 4 | 5 to 6 | 5 to 6 | 4 or more |
| 20-54 years | 2 | 6 to 7 | 5 to 6 | 4 or more |
| 55 years and over | 2 | 5 to 6 | 5 to 6 | 4 or more |

**Table 5.11   Weekly Menu Planning Chart**

| | Sunday | Monday | Tuesday | Wednesday | Thursday | Friday | Saturday |
|---|---|---|---|---|---|---|---|
| **Breakfast**<br>Fruit<br>Cereal<br>Entree<br>Bread<br>Beverage | | | | | | | |
| **Lunch**<br>Soup (optional)<br>Protein Entree<br>Vegetable or Salad<br>Bread<br>Fruit (optional)<br>Dessert (optional)<br>Beverage | | | | | | | |
| **Dinner**<br>Soup or Salad<br>(optional)<br>Protein Entree<br>Vegetables<br>Bread<br>Fruit<br>Dessert (optional)<br>Beverage | | | | | | | |
| **Snacks** | | | | | | | |

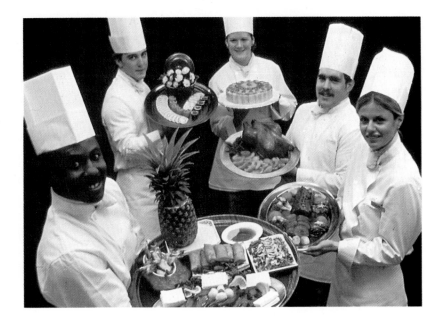

***Figure 5.9.*** Color, flavor, texture, and nutrient content all contribute to an attractive, enjoyable meal.

## Table 5.12    Sample Grocery List Format

| Food Group Category | Form | Amount to Buy |
|---|---|---|
| Milk Products: | | |
| Protein Foods: | | |
| Fruits and Vegetables: | | |
| Breads and Cereals: | | |
| Fats and Oils: | | |
| Miscellaneous: | | |

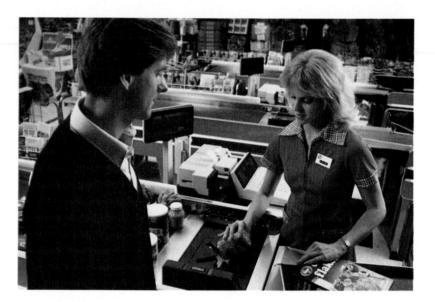

***Figure 5.10.*** Shopping for groceries requires a good deal of self-restraint.

***Money-Saving Tips.*** After the food budget has been determined and the meals have been planned, it is time to go grocery shopping. A trip to the grocery store is an exercise in self-restraint! Marketing strategies often encourage you to buy more of a product, or perhaps unnecessary products. The aisle arrangement, product placement on shelves, lighting, and color scheme can be hidden persuaders in food selection. The following are a few consumer survival tips:

- Complete a grocery list and stick to it
- Check newspaper foods ads for special prices
- Shop once a week to avoid impulse buying

***Illustration 5.3.*** Unit Pricing Helps Determine the Best Buy.

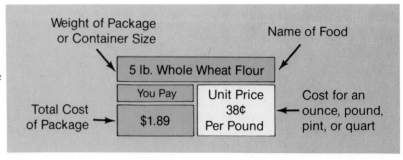

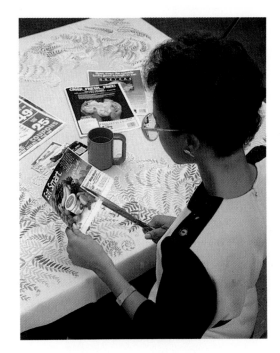

*Figure 5.11.* Coupons can be cost-cutters if they are used wisely.

- Compare prices at various types of food stores, such as a supermarket chain, convenience store, corner grocery, and warehouse market
- Shop on a full stomach
- Use *unit pricing* (the price per ounce or pound) to determine the best buy (See Illustration 5.3)
- Compare the costs of *generic* (no company identified on the product) and *brand name* (label of major food company) products
- Use coupons if they are for items you use regularly and if the reduced price is less than that of other brands
- Limit the purchase of foods with a low nutrient density

Depending on location, shopping at more than one store may save money. Supermarkets offer a large variety and generally feature specials. Convenience stores and specialty shops are usually more expensive. Buying larger quantities of staples, canned items, and frozen foods once a month at a food warehouse is also economical for larger households. Before buying large amounts of any item, consider

## Table 5.13   Storage of Meat and Poultry

| Product | Refrigerator (days at 40° F) | Freezer (months at 0° F) |
|---|---|---|
| **Fresh Meats** | | |
| Roasts (Beef) | 3 to 5 | 6 to 12 |
| Roasts (Lamb) | 3 to 5 | 6 to 9 |
| Roasts (Pork, Veal) | 3 to 5 | 4 to 8 |
| Steaks (Beef) | 3 to 5 | 6 to 12 |
| Chops (Lamb) | 3 to 5 | 6 to 9 |
| Chops (Pork) | 3 to 5 | 3 to 4 |
| Hamburger, Ground and Stew Meats | 1 to 2 | 3 to 4 |
| Variety Meats (Tongue, Brain, Kidneys, Liver, and Heart) | 1 to 2 | 3 to 4 |
| Sausage (Pork) | 1 to 2 | 1 to 2 |
| **Cooked Meats** | | |
| Cooked Meat and Meat Dishes | 3 to 4 | 2 to 3 |
| Gravy and Meat Broth | 1 to 2 | 2 to 3 |
| **Processed Meats**[a] | | |
| Bacon | 7 | 1 |
| Frankfurters | 7[b] | 1 to 2 |
| Ham (whole) | 7 | 1 to 2 |
| Ham (half) | 3 to 5 | 1 to 2 |
| Ham (slices) | 3 to 4 | 1 to 2 |
| Luncheon meats | 3 to 5[b] | 1 to 2 |
| Sausage (smoked) | 7 | 1 to 2 |
| Sausage (dry, semi-dry) | 14 to 21 | 1 to 2 |
| **Fresh Poultry** | | |
| Chicken and Turkey (whole) | 1 to 2 | 12 |
| Chicken pieces | 1 to 2 | 9 |
| Turkey pieces | 1 to 2 | 6 |

Source: United States Department of Agriculture, Food Safety and Inspection Service, "The Safe Food Book: Your Kitchen Guide" (Washington, D.C.: United States Government Printing Office, 1984), Home and Garden Bulletin No. 241.

[a]Frozen, cured meat loses quality rapidly and should be used as soon as possible.

[b]Once a vacuum-sealed package is opened. Unopened vacuum-sealed packages can be stored in the refrigerator for 2 weeks.

## Table 5.13 (cont'd)

| Product | Refrigerator (days at 40° F) | Freezer (months at 0° F) |
|---|---|---|
| **Fresh Poultry (cont'd)** | | |
| Duck and Goose (whole) | 1 to 2 | 6 |
| Giblets | 1 to 2 | 3 to 4 |
| **Cooked Poultry** | | |
| Covered with Broth, Gravy | 1 to 2 | 6 |
| Pieces not in Broth or Gravy | 3 to 4 | 1 |
| Cooked Poultry dishes | 3 to 4 | 4 to 6 |
| Fried Chicken | 3 to 4 | 4 |
| **Game** | | |
| Deer | 3 to 5 | 6 to 12 |
| Rabbit | 1 to 2 | 12 |
| Duck and Goose (whole, wild) | 1 to 2 | 6 |

storage space, quantity normally used, and shelf-life of the product. Savings from quantity buying may be lost by food spoilage. On the other hand, making frequent trips to a grocery store can be time consuming and costly.

*Food Storage.* An important task after shopping is the correct storage of the food purchased. Perishable items should be refrigerated or frozen. See Table 5.13. Make certain that meat is wrapped well before storage. Avoid contact between raw and cooked foods to assure food safety. Store fresh vegetables and greens in a moisture-controlled container, such as a hydrator or crisper. Store staples, such as flour and sugar, at room temperature in a container with a lid to keep out insects. Canned goods should be stored in a dry, clean cupboard. Always place newly purchased items at the back of the cupboard, so that older items are used first.

*Preparing Meals.* Meal preparation also requires planning. Some items may need to be taken out of the freezer the night before meal preparation. Other items will require preparation in advance. *Check the recipe ahead of time.* The most challenging part of meal

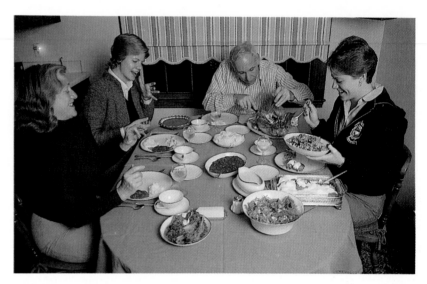

*Figure 5.12.* Successful meal planning and preparation will result in a nutritious meal everyone will enjoy.

preparation is getting all the food done at the same time; knowing what task must be started first is essential. The quality of many hot foods can decrease rapidly if they are held for any length of time. It may be helpful to work backward in planning the schedule. Decide the time the meal is to be served, then check recipes for total preparation time needed. Experience will aid in judging the time it takes to prepare various recipes. Also, be prepared to be flexible as circumstances change. For example, a friend may stop for a visit at meal time. Is there enough food for you and your friend, or will the menu have to be changed?

## Evaluate Your Results

Once you've had some experience, evaluate your results. Ask the following questions to judge your degree of success:

- Are the meals nutritious?
- Did you stay within the food budget?
- Was there adequate food available for everyone?
- Were the meals appetizing and attractively served?
- Did the meals require more preparation time than expected?

- Was any food wasted or allowed to spoil?
- Were clean-up tasks completed?

## Feedback

Feedback on success of the plan is an important part of the process. Effective communication between household members improves the likelihood of success in food management.

# SKILL BUILDING FOR A HEALTHIER YOU

First, you mastered the basics of nutritional science. Now you have identified the tools for nutrition survival in the marketplace. The next task is to understand the factors that influence your nutritional needs and food choices. This understanding enables you to control your food decisions.

## CHECK YOUR PROGRESS

1. Describe the purpose of a food guide.
2. List the five food groups identified in the Hassle-Free Guide to a Better Diet.
3. Identify the meal planning tool used in planning diabetic or Calorie-controlled diets.
4. Name the joint United States Department of Agriculture and Department of Health and Human Services publication that suggests dietary modifications for the American public. Why were these guidelines developed?
5. Are all foods within each food group equally good sources of a given nutrient? Cite several examples to support your answer.
6. What are some of the reasons for differences in the nutrient values of foods? How does a baked potato differ from potato chips?
7. What is meant by nutrient density? How is a value calculated?

8. How can food processing change the calorie and nutrient content of food?
9. Identify the tool available for consumers to use in comparing nutritional value of food products. What is the basis for the U.S. RDA?
10. What are the four steps in planning meals and snacks? Identify key questions to ask during each step.
11. Identify several practices that can help a consumer save money at the grocery store.

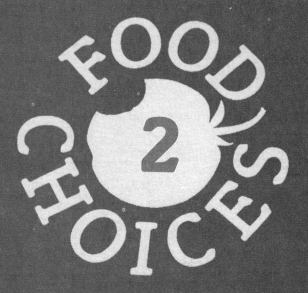

**FOOD CHOICES**

2

## MAKING INFORMED DECISIONS